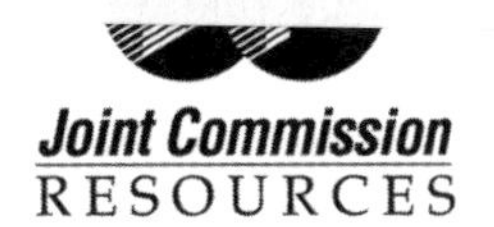

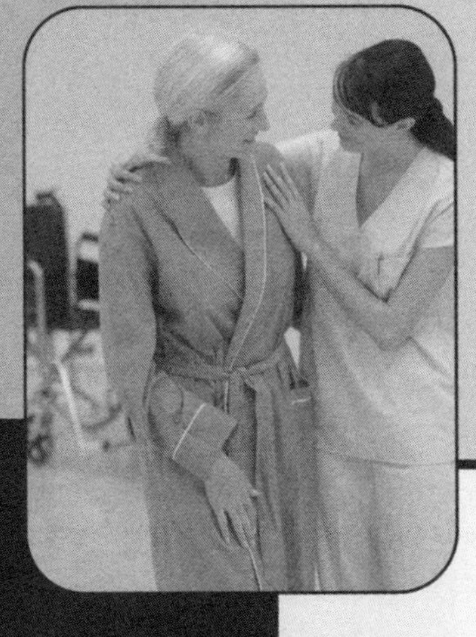

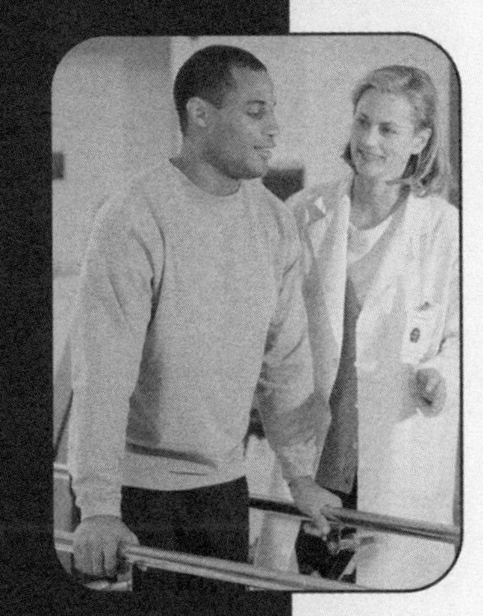

REDUCING THE RISK OF FALLS *in Your Health Care Organization*

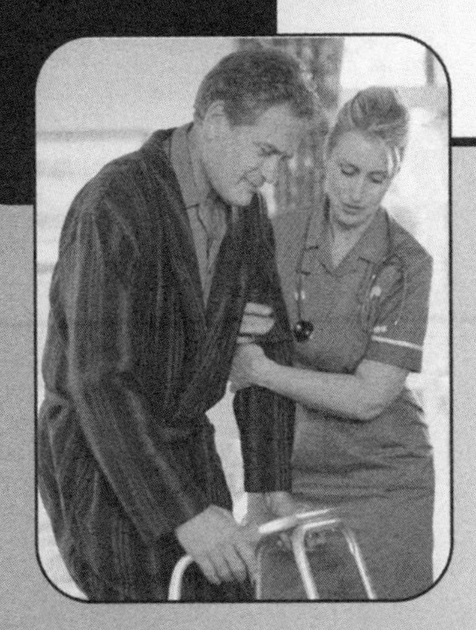

Improving Health Care Quality and Safety

REDUCING THE RISK OF FALLS *in Your Health Care Organization*

Editor: Ilese J. Smith
Project Manager: Cheryl Firestone
Manager, Publications: Eileen Norris
Production Manager: Johanna Harris
Associate Director: Cecily Pew
Executive Director: Catherine Chopp Hinckley
Vice President, Publications: George J. Farina
Joint Commission/JCR Reviewers: Marianna Grachek, M.S.N., C.N.H.A., C.A.L.A.; Jean Rose-DeRenzy, R.N., M.S., C.N.R.N.; Carol Ally, R.N., B.S.N.; Madhavi Davé, R.N., M.S.N., M.B.A.; Diane Kucic, R.N., B.S., C.P.H.Q.; Carol Ptasinski, R.N., M.S.N., M.B.A.; Rosemarie Savino, R.N., B.S.N.; Mary Schleinzer, R.N., B.S.N., M.S.

Joint Commission Resources Mission
The mission of Joint Commission Resources is to continuously improve the safety and quality of care in the United States and in the international community through the provision of education and consultation services and international accreditation.

Joint Commission Resources educational programs and publications support, but are separate from, the accreditation activities of the Joint Commission. Attendees at Joint Commission Resources educational programs and purchasers of Joint Commission Resources publications receive no special consideration or treatment in, or confidential information about, the accreditation process.

Joint Commission Resources, Inc. (JCR), a not-for-profit affiliate of the Joint Commission on Accreditation of Healthcare Organizations (Joint Commission), has been designated by the Joint Commission to publish publications and multimedia products. JCR reproduces and distributes these materials under license from the Joint Commission.

Printed in the U.S.A. 5 4 3 2 1

Requests for permission to make copies of any part of this work should be mailed to
Permissions Editor
Department of Publications
Joint Commission Resources
One Renaissance Boulevard
Oakbrook Terrace, Illinois 60181
permissions@jcrinc.com

ISBN: 0-86688-942-6
Library of Congress Control Number: 20059238500

For more information about Joint Commission Resources, please visit http://www.jcrinc.com.

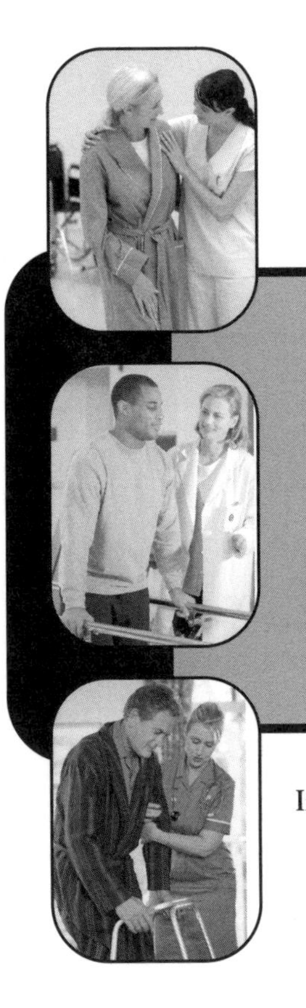

TABLE OF CONTENTS

Introduction 1

A Culture of Safety 1

A Note on Terminology 4

Acknowledgments 4

Chapter 1: Defining the Problem of Falls 13

Defining Falls 14

The Frequency of Falls 14

Classifying Falls and Fall Risk 15

Common Causes of Falls 18

The Physical Costs of Falls 19

The Financial Costs of Falls 21

Joint Commission Requirements Related to Falls 22

Chapter 2: Strategies for Addressing the Root Causes of Falls 29

Tracking the Root Causes of Falls 30

Root Cause Cases and Intervention Strategies 32

Root Cause Example: Inadequate Caregiver Communication 32

Root Cause Example: Inadequate Staff Orientation and Training 33

Root Cause Example: Inadequate Assessment and Reassessment 35

Root Cause Example: Unsafe Environment of Care 38

Root Cause Examples: Inadequate Care Planning and Provision 41

(continued)

Chapter 3: The Elements of Effective Fall Risk Assessment 51
A Team Approach to Risk Assessment 52
Strokes as a Risk Factor 62
Multiple Risk Factors. 62
Categorizing Risk Assessment Tools. 65
Choosing the Appropriate Assessment Tool 66
Measuring the Progress of Risk Assessment 70

Chapter 4: Establishing a Fall Reduction Program 81
The Principles of a Fall Reduction Program. 82
The Principles of Intervention 84
Interventions for All Care Recipients. 87
Individual Interventions for High-Risk Care Recipients 91
Approaches to Care Recipient Lifting and Repositioning. 94
Interventions That Maintain an Individualized Approach 99
Interventions Supported by Research and Decision Making 100
Collecting and Using Data in Developing Interventions 104
Consistent Documentation in the Intervention Process. 105
Institutional Support for Interventions 112

Chapter 5: Measuring Success of a Fall Reduction Program. 117
Necessary Steps Toward Measuring Program Effectiveness. 117
Analyzing the Data to Measure Progress 120
Comparing Data to Reduce Falls and Measure Results 124
Performance Data Standards for Improvement 126
The Joint Commission Staffing Effectiveness Standard 131
Drawing Conclusions on Fall Reduction Programs 132

Glossary 145

Index 151

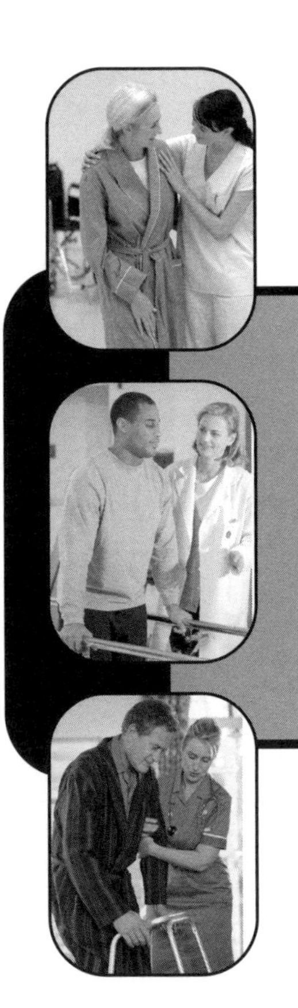

INTRODUCTION

A Culture of Safety

In recent years, health care organizations have paid increasing attention to the atmosphere in which they provide care. The term *a culture of safety* has become a familiar buzzword to organizations that have come to realize the positive impact a healthy and open organizational culture can make on improving care. An atmosphere of mutual trust in which staff members can talk freely about safety problems and how to solve them, without fear of negative consequences, is now seen as essential to improving safety in any organization.

The issue of falls is one primary safety concern that organizations must take into account when attempting to improve their internal culture. It has been reported that falls are the single most significant adverse event experienced in hospitals. Aside from the obvious and immediate injuries that can result from a fall, these incidents can also have an affect on long-term function, physical and emotional health, independence, and quality of life. In many cases, a fall also leads to an extended length of stay and increases the risk of another fall.[1]

Although this book looks specifically at the problem of falls by examining various risk assessment tools, intervention strategies, steps toward establishing a fall reduction program, and the measuring techniques involved in the process, it does so with a perspective that takes into account the increasing focus on improving safety culture.

This positive trend has resulted in an increased interest in safety culture assessment in health care organizations. Culture assessment tools offer organizations the opportunity to analyze and understand the atmosphere of their settings in order to consider plans for transformation. Many health care organizations have been motivated to initiate safety culture assessments to fulfill directives that come from a membership in a larger health care system, consortium, or payer groups with a stake in providing safe health care service.

Other health care organizations are undertaking safety culture assessments to provide regulatory agencies with evidence of their patient or resident safety activities, or as one way of fulfilling Joint Commission standards. Safety culture assessment is not a specific mandate, but the Joint Commission does require organizations that collect data to monitor performance, including data on staff opinions and needs, staff willingness to report medical or health care errors, perceptions of risks to patients and residents, and suggestions for improving safety. Below is the Joint Commission 2006 National Patient Safety Goal on fall reduction for applicable settings.

Fall Reduction Goal

Goal: Reduce the risk of patient/resident harm resulting from falls.

Requirement: Implement a fall reduction program and evaluate the effectiveness of the program. (Applicable to the following programs: Assisted Living, Critical Access Hospitals, Home Care, Hospitals, and Long Term Care.)

The issues explored in the chapters ahead are interwoven with corroborating assertions that a culture of safety is essential to any initiative to improve safety.

Chapter 1: *Defining the Problem of Falls* begins by outlining both the physical and financial costs of care recipient falls. Offering expert analysis and recognized research studies, it also defines and classifies falls as a way of identifying risk factors and reduction strategies in different care settings. In reviewing the assessment requirements that health care institutions are bound by, it provides a solid foundation for an organizational culture and the recommended procedures that guide institutions toward more effective reduction measures.

Chapter 2: *Strategies for Addressing the Root Causes of Falls* employs a series of examples in investigating specific causes and determining potential avenues of reduction in each case. The root causes explored and discussed all center around the organizational culture and include unsafe environment of care; inadequate caregiver communication; inadequate assessment and reassessment; inadequate care planning and provision; and inadequate staffing, orientation, training, and supervision.

Chapter 3: *The Elements of Effective Fall Risk Assessment* delves into perhaps the most important aspect of a successful fall reduction program. It begins by outlining the significance of taking a team approach toward risk assessment and offers a variety of baseline tips to consider in implementing proper methods. It both categorizes assessment tools and offers guidelines for selecting appropriate assessment tools. It closely examines the essentials of managing the process of assessment and offers suggestions on approaches designed to help measure the progress of risk assessment programs.

Chapter 4: *Establishing a Fall Reduction Program* begins with a broad characterization of the fundamental aspects and challenges of establishing a fall reduction program. By classifying reduction strategies and reviewing environmental interventions, this chapter helps chart a course for implementing systemwide intervention plans, communication policies, and transfer protocols. The chapter also stresses the importance of maintaining an individualized approach by focusing on individual interventions for high-risk patients and residents, as well as establishing indicators and interventions for those with mobility problems. Using validated reports and case studies, it clearly illustrates that an effective fall reduction program relies on the strength of research and decision making, consistent documentation, proper methods of collecting and using data, and institutional support that is proactive and ongoing.

Chapter 5: *Measuring Success of a Fall Reduction Program* looks at the structures that need to be in place for a health care organization to effectively measure the plan and progress of its fall reduction program. Offering guidelines for performance improvement and for analyzing data and determining appropriate measures and indicators, this chapter focuses on assessing overall outcomes in the effort to reduce falls.

According to the Institute of Medicine, "*the biggest challenge to moving toward a safer health system is changing the culture from one of blaming individuals for errors to one in which errors are treated not as personal failures, but as opportunities to improve the system and prevent harm.*"[2]

There is a growing understanding in the health care industry that a variety of factors—from the emphasis on production and cost controls[3], to organizational and individual inability to acknowledge fallibility[4] among health care providers[5]—combine to create a culture contradictory to the requirements of safety. It is these factors that form a culture in which the health care industry itself is viewed as a potential risk factor to the very individuals it serves.

In an article titled "Safety Culture Assessment: A Tool for Improving Patient Safety in Health Care Organizations," authors V.F. Nieva and J. Sorra suggest the following:

Professional and organizational cultures in health care must undergo a transformation in the interest of promoting safer care. Health care must come to see itself as a high hazard industry which is inherently risky. It must abandon the philosophy of requiring perfect, error free performance from individuals and focus, instead, on designing systems for safety. Health care systems must move away from the current "blame and shame" culture that prevents acknowledgement of error and therefore obstructs any possibility of learning from error. Safety improvement requires that health care systems have ready access to information that supports learning from experience in order to promote systems that both prevent errors and mitigate the impact of errors that occur. In contrast to a "pathological culture" where failure is punished or concealed and people refuse to acknowledge that problems exist, a positive safety culture recognizes the inevitability of error and proactively seeks to identify latent threats.[6]

The article also supports the belief that a health care organization's ability to reach its potential will be realized only when it is able to create a culture of safety among its staff. This, of course, is achievable only if the organization views patient and resident safety as one of its highest priorities.

Nieva and Sorra's work also includes brief examples from organizations that have undertaken such assessments and that take a sharper look at critical processes that need to be considered when deciding to use safety culture assessment tools. Portions of this article are included in Sidebar I-1, beginning on page 5.

There is no mistaking the need for reduction of risks associated with patient and resident falls throughout the health care industry. For any health care organization considering establishing, improving, or redesigning a comprehensive fall program, success likely begins with a thorough assessment of its organizational culture.

Readers may want to think about the principles, strategies, and tools described in this book as they are applicable to real-world experiences and as they are presented to accommodate flexibility within every kind of health care organization. Ultimately, it is the goal of the health care industry to protect the care recipient, as well as those who provide care.

A Note on Terminology

Throughout this book, the words *care recipient, patient,* or *resident* are used to describe the person, client, or consumer who actually receives health care services.

Acknowledgments

We would like to express our sincere appreciation to the individuals and health care organizations that allowed us to include information about fall reduction methods and programs in this book. A special thank-you is extended to Dave Whitaker for his outstanding job in writing this book.

References

1. Wilson E.B.: Preventing patient falls. *AACN Clinical Issues* 9:100–108, 1998.
2. Institute of Medicine: *Crossing the quality chasm: A new health system for the 21st century.* Washington, DC: National Academy Press, 2001.
3. Gaba D.M., Howard S.K., Jump B.: Production pressure in the work environment. California anesthesiologists' attitudes and experiences: *Anesthesiology* 81:488–500, 1994.
4. Leape L.L.: Error in medicine. *JAMA* 272:1851–1857, 1994.
5. Krizek T.J.: Surgical error: Ethical issues of adverse events. *Arch Surg* 135:1359–1366, 2000.
6. Nieva V.F., Sorra J.: Safety culture assessment: A tool for improving patient safety in healthcare organizations. Agency for Healthcare Research and Quality, Department of Health and Human Services. 2004. http://www.ahrq.gov (accessed Feb. 10, 2005).

SIDEBAR I-1

Culture Assessment Tools

The Advisory Committee on the Safety of Nuclear Installations provides the following definition of safety culture that can easily be adapted to the context of safety in health care:

> The safety culture of an organization is the product of individual and group values, attitudes, perceptions, competencies, and patterns of behavior that determine the commitment to, and the style and proficiency of, an organization's health and safety management. Organizations with a positive safety culture are characterized by communications founded on mutual trust, by shared perceptions of the importance of safety, and by confidence in the efficacy of preventive measures.

The conceptual breadth of the safety culture concept illustrated in this definition is reflected in the wide range of topics covered by safety culture assessment instruments. These instruments often assess the values, attitudes, behaviors, and norms of organization members. They may also focus on perceptions of the organizational context, such as managerial priorities, adequacy of training and resources, or policies and procedures.

An important characteristic of safety culture assessment tools is whether they take a managerial or staff perspective, or combine elements of both. Some measurement tools focus on management assessments of safety policies and practices in their organizations. These tools assess managerial perspectives about what they see as occurring or needing to occur in their organizations, as represented by formal policies and standard operating practices. These instruments are intended to provide the leadership in health care organizations with information about the status of official organizational practices, to generate awareness about safety practices, and to motivate them to take action in areas needing improvement.

An example of a management self-assessment tool focused on safety was developed by VHA (previously known as Voluntary Hospitals of America) in conjunction with the American Hospital Association (AHA) titled *Strategies for Leadership: An Organizational Approach to Patient Safety*. The instrument is intended to be used by multidisciplinary teams, including both direct-care providers and middle and top managers in hospital settings. Items are organized according to key safety aspects such as patient safety as a leadership priority, promoting a nonpunitive culture for sharing information, fostering teamwork, routinely assessing the risk of errors and adverse events, and involving patients and families in care delivery. For each key aspect, managers are asked to respond to statements that describe pertinent activities using a five-point scale to indicate the extent to which the activity has been implemented throughout the organization (from "there has been no discussion around this activity," to "this activity is fully implemented throughout the organization"). Examples of statements used to assess one of the key aspects in this assessment tool, "promotion of a nonpunitive culture," are shown below.

Management items to measure promotion of a nonpunitive culture include the following:

- The organization has a nonpunitive policy to address patient adverse events, including medical staff and organization employees.

(continued)

SIDEBAR I-1 (continued)

- The activity of legal counsel is aligned with the patient safety agenda to ensure consumer, public, and legal accountability while concurrently protecting the organization.
- Leadership encourages and rewards recognition and reporting of adverse events and near misses.

Other safety culture assessment tools focus on staff perceptions and attitudes. Rather than eliciting the views of senior managers, these instruments focus on perceptions of what occurs in the daily life of the organization from the perspective of direct patient-care providers and other staff who have an impact on patient safety. These tools belong to a long tradition of quantitative organizational culture and climate assessments in health care and safety culture studies in a variety of high-risk industries such as offshore oil drilling, air traffic control, aircraft carrier maintenance, and manufacturing.

These staff-based assessments are structured self-report surveys that elicit perceptions of the working environment from the perspective of staff at the "sharp end" of health care delivery in various settings (for example, emergency rooms, intensive care units, hospitals, nursing homes, ambulatory care clinics). Typically, health care staff are asked to respond to a list of descriptive statements that are designed to operationalize various safety culture domains. Respondents indicate their agreement (for example, from "strongly disagree" to "strongly agree") or the frequency with which events described occur (for example, from "never" to "always"). Examples of items in these staff-based assessment tools are shown below.

Items in staff-based culture assessment instruments include the following:

- When a mistake is discovered, we try to figure out what problems in the work process led to the mistake.
- Supervisors and employees discuss how to handle incidents involving error.
- Employees may believe that event reports are held against them.

These instruments derive numerical scores that indicate the type of culture characterizing the organization, such as a group oriented or hierarchical culture. Scores may also be used to indicate the organization's standing on multiple culture domains such as openness of communication, teamwork, or perceptions of event reporting. The scores can be calculated at different levels of aggregation: the organization as a whole, organizational units (departments, clinical areas, hospital wings or floors), or different professional groups (physicians, nurses, or laboratory staff).

Much research is currently under way to develop and use safety culture assessment tools. For example, in 2000 the U.S. Veterans Health Administration (VHA), part of the U.S. Department of Veterans Affairs (VA) launched a large-scale effort to measure prevailing beliefs and behavior surrounding safety and errors in all VA hospitals. At the University of Texas, patient safety researchers have developed a number of related assessment instruments adapted from aviation crew resource management measures to study cultures within various hospital units. Between 2000 and 2003, the Agency for Healthcare Research and Quality funded more than 100 patient safety research grants and contracts. A number of these research projects use or have developed safety culture and organizational culture assessment tools.

(continued)

SIDEBAR I-1 (continued)

Implementing a safety culture assessment involves the commitment of staff time and resources. Why do health care organizations decide to assess safety culture? How are the data used? The answers to these questions can be good predictors of the extent to which culture data eventually contribute to real patient safety improvement in an institution.

Health care organizations may conduct safety culture assessments for a variety of reasons, but they are not mutually exclusive and, indeed, can often occur in combination. Culture assessments can be used to: (1) diagnose safety culture to identify areas for improvement and raise awareness about patient safety; (2) evaluate patient safety interventions or programs and track change over time; (3) conduct internal and external benchmarking; and (4) fulfill directives or regulatory requirements.

Diagnosing Safety Culture and Raising Awareness
A safety culture assessment provides an organization with a basic understanding of the safety-related perceptions and attitudes of its managers and staff. Safety culture measures can be used as diagnostic tools to identify areas for improvement. A safety culture assessment can help an organization identify areas that are considered more problematic than others because there are many potential starting points for improvement efforts. Cultural issues that are identified as problematic can provide material for further analysis of underlying "root causes" and for generating improvement ideas from staff directly involved in the issues.

Safety culture assessment can also launch an organization's patient safety program. Assessing patient safety culture has a corollary effect, intended or not, of raising awareness levels about the role of culture in promoting a safer patient environment. Assessments communicate what is important to an organization, what are desirable end states, and what factors are viewed as leading to those end states. Safety culture assessments can function as symbolic communications that focus attention on cultural priorities and establish a common vocabulary and set of goals to rally behind. In this way, assessment in itself may be regarded as a patient safety intervention.

Evaluating Safety Interventions or Programs and Tracking Change over Time
Changes in safety culture can be used as evidence of the effectiveness of patient safety programs and interventions. In this context, culture change is regarded as an "outcome measure," usually in conjunction with more direct measures of patient safety, such as error rates and clinical outcomes. Safety culture assessments provide a way of tracking progress in cultural transformation over time. Baseline measures of culture can be taken before intervention is implemented, with follow-up measures after the intervention is underway. The scale of these assessments and the frequency with which they are conducted will differ, depending on the program or intervention under evaluation.

Safety culture change is currently being tracked as part of several large-scale patient safety programs. Baseline culture measures have been taken in the VHA, and periodic assessments are planned in the future as part of an ambitious patient safety program that includes a patient safety reporting and analysis system, technology usability assessments, and

(continued)

SIDEBAR I-1 (continued)

methodologies for prioritizing safety-related actions. Johns Hopkins Hospital is using safety culture measures, among others, to assess the impact of interventions implemented within their comprehensive patient safety program—including patient safety education; an active multidisciplinary safety committee that reviews the hospital's programs, policies and procedures; and executive walk around.

In organizations with ongoing patient safety improvement programs, periodic safety culture measurements can be used to refine changes in repeated Plan-Do-Study-Act (PDSA) cycles. A continuing measurement effort can be used as part of a formative evaluation effort that is an integral part of a safety improvement program. Optimally, safety culture assessments would become part of an organizational learning and continuous improvement process.

Conducting Internal and External Benchmarking

Theoretically, safety culture assessments can be used to compare units within one organization or to examine differences across different organizations or systems. Such benchmarking comparisons have grown in popularity in the quality improvement and consumer empowerment movements in various settings, including health care. Internal benchmarking can be conducted with relative ease when a culture assessment tool is used across the various departments and clinical areas of a health care organization. Often, data are provided to unit managers, comparing their specific information with data from the entire organization.

External benchmarking is technically possible when a common assessment tool is used across many organizations. Benchmarked data can be used by health care consumers choosing health care delivery organizations, and by the organizations' quality improvement and competitor analysis efforts. For example, in the United States, the National Committee for Quality Assurance publishes the Quality Compass, which provides national, regional, and individual health plan data on performance (Health Plan Employer Data and Information Set: HEDIS) and customer satisfaction (Consumer Assessments of Health Plans: CAHPs). Report cards about hospitals provide consumers with comparative data on customer satisfaction and various aspects of care. In Canada, for example, the Ontario Hospital Association and the government of Ontario collaborated to produce "Hospital Report 2002: Acute Care," which presents comparative data for 92 acute care hospitals.

Clearly, health care organizations are interested in the potential for benchmarking as they decide to undertake safety culture assessments. However, organizational culture assessments are in the early stages of development; whether the data can actually be consolidated and standardized to the point of being useful for external benchmarking remains to be seen.

Selecting a Safety Culture Assessment Tool

To achieve maximal benefit from conducting a safety culture assessment, health care organizations must attend to several critical processes—from involving key stakeholders to planning safety improvements based on the data. These are critical processes because they are potential stumbling blocks for organizations attempting to use safety culture assessment as a tool for patient safety improvement.

(continued)

SIDEBAR I-1 (continued)

When the rationale and objectives for a safety culture assessment have been clarified and all key stakeholders have been consulted, a safety culture assessment tool must be selected or developed. We recommend that health care organizations first examine the suitability of existing tools to their needs before embarking on an effort to develop a new tool. Criteria for suitability include: (1) the domains of culture that are assessed, (2) the types of staff who are expected to complete the tool, (3) the settings for which the tool was developed, and (4) the availability of reliability and validity evidence about the tool.

It is important to select a tool that best suits the purposes for which the data will be used and that covers the aspects of culture that are of interest to the organization. If the goal is to obtain a summary view of the status of patient safety culture, an instrument that covers a few major safety topics might suffice. If the purpose is more diagnostic with the intent of identifying areas that may present high risks for patient harm, a tool that covers a broader range of safety culture areas would offer more value. To evaluate the effects of a specific patient safety intervention it is important to choose a tool that measures the specific cultural domains that will be affected.

The intended source of information for the tools—senior managers; specific types of staff such as nurses, pharmacists, or physicians; or all staff types and levels—should also be checked for suitability. Tools designed for senior managers may address issues about which other staff are typically uninformed, or may elicit information specifically geared toward a management perspective. Similarly, tools designed for nurses may not address safety culture issues that reflect the concerns of physicians or administrative managers. Safety culture assessment tools are also typically targeted for specific settings. For example, some tools may focus on safety culture issues specific to hospitals. Others may focus on pharmacies, ambulatory facilities, nursing homes, or intensive care units. Modification may be required when adopting a tool for a setting other than the one for which it was intended.

Information about the quality of culture assessment tools is currently difficult to find. Evidence on instrument reliability is lacking for many, and validity evidence is even more elusive. Like other patient safety improvement tools, there is limited evidence establishing a linkage between positive safety culture and positive clinical outcomes or medical error reduction. However, some studies have shown linkages between staff perceptions of culture and outcomes such as quality of care and lower risk adjusted length of stay. A strong safety climate has also been found to be associated with compliance with safety work practices among nurses. As more safety culture assessments are done, more validity evidence related to culture assessment is expected.

For health care organizations, the search for an existing safety culture assessment tool that can meet all their needs can be challenging. Although a number of tools have been developed, many are not readily accessible. Some safety culture tools are proprietary and are only available for a fee. Published research studies that use safety culture assessment tools typically do not include the full instrument; copies must be requested through the primary author. Unpublished tools can be even more difficult to locate.

(continued)

SIDEBAR I-1 (continued)

Recent reviews of quantitative measures of safety culture and organizational culture in health care provide good information about published culture assessment tools. These reviews outline the dimensions assessed, the settings in which they have been administered, the number of items, and information about their reliability and validity. However, these reviews do not include the many proprietary and unpublished tools that are available or that have recently been developed and are currently being used in health care organizations. Ideally, it would be very useful to have an inventory that lists both published and unpublished safety culture assessment tools that have been developed, including information on their technical specifications, usage, and contact information to obtain review copies. For now, however, the process of locating safety culture assessment tools to consider using will require effort and time.

Using Effective Data Collection Procedures

Collecting safety culture assessment data typically involves the use of survey administration methods. Although numerous texts provide guidelines on classic survey methodologies and their application to organizational settings—for example, sampling, advance communication, follow-up to maximize response rates, preventing bias in data—it is not uncommon for these procedures to be overlooked by staff conducting assessments in health care organizations.

When procedures to collect assessment data are not well designed, the quantity, quality, and generalized ability of the data are likely to be negatively affected. Health care organizations risk obtaining assessment data that, in the end, may prove to be unusable. Response rates frequently suffer due to inadequate preparation. In one extreme case in an urban community hospital, only one staff member completed the culture assessment over a two-day period. Staff were asked to go to a designated room to complete the assessment, but inadequate advance notification and staff concerns about data confidentiality were thought to have led to the lack of response. Sometimes the use of new technologies for data collection that are successful in some settings may be ill-advised in health care organizations. For example, a number of health care researchers have been unable to achieve adequate responses using Web-based assessment tools due to the limited access of hospital employees to computers with online connections.

Procedures that result in inaccurate or biased data may be even more serious because they are harder to detect. For example, one national health care system instructed some of its member hospitals to have staff complete a safety culture assessment tool after viewing a videotape promoting patient safety. It is likely that staff responses to the assessment were affected by the priming effect of the video. In addition, each hospital was instructed to obtain at least 50 completed surveys. But because no guidance was provided on sampling procedures, it is not possible to determine the representativeness of the data.

Health care organizations collecting their own assessment data should become knowledgeable about survey administration procedure scenarios like these. Organizations should not underestimate the knowledge and level of effort that is required not only to collect the data, but to analyze and synthesize the results. Failure to attend to these processes can seriously affect the outcomes of an assessment effort.

(continued)

SIDEBAR I-1 (continued)

Implementing an Action Plan and Initiating Change

If a safety culture assessment reveals a punitive culture that suppresses adverse event reporting, how does an organization move from these data to usable knowledge, and from knowledge to sustainable change? The effectiveness of safety culture data as a tool for patient safety improvement requires processes for developing a shared organizational understanding of the underlying meanings and causes of the data, and for identifying the range of potential actions relevant to those interpretations. Rather than viewing the assessment results as an end point, the information should be considered the starting point from which action and patient safety changes emerge.

Practitioners in data-based cultural transformation, organizational change, and continuous quality improvement discuss the importance of using a systematic process involving data feedback, problem solving, action planning, and monitoring to facilitate the progression from data to action. Results are typically provided to top managers after a culture assessment, but one of the most common complaints from employees who participate in these assessments is the lack of feedback about the results and any subsequent improvement actions. If safety culture assessments are to lead to culture change, feedback should be provided to all who contribute to the assessment. Results can be presented by organization or facility, by unit or team, by staff categories, or by other groupings relevant to the purposes of the assessment. In this way, assessment data can be used for localized patient safety improvement efforts at various levels and sections of the organization.

For greater impact, feedback can be combined with action planning sessions. These sessions have been shown to be most effective when they are conducted by trained line managers rather than top management, external experts, or specialized staff. In health care organizations, clinical staff, departmental managers, and supervisors must be involved in leading feedback discussions, not just delegating these functions to specialized staff in the quality improvement, patient safety, or risk management departments. The fruitfulness of the data utilization process can rest heavily on the skill of the session leaders. In the hands of naïve facilitators, sessions can easily deteriorate into unproductive defensiveness and negativism. Because facilitation and action planning require specialized skills, health care managers and clinicians should be provided with specific training and action planning aids to enable them to be comfortable and effective in these roles.

Feedback and action planning sessions are typically conducted in groups that have been assembled for this specific purpose. These groups are designed in different ways, depending on the nature of the organization and its goals. Feedback and action planning sessions must be designed with care, bringing together multidisciplinary groups while recognizing the complexities of health care organizations and their dual clinical and administrative authority structures.

Assessment data are likely to point to many different areas of culture that could be improved, accompanied by different interpretations about potential actions that could be taken in each

(continued)

SIDEBAR I-1 (continued)

area. Incremental changes can be implemented and tested on a small scale, changing one process or practice at a time, in only particular units of the organization, or over a short trial period. Improvements in aviation safety over the years have relied on the widespread implementation of hundreds of small changes in procedures, equipment, training, and organization that aggregated to establish effective practices and a strong safety culture. In patient safety, as in aviation, there is no one "silver bullet."

Safety culture assessments are new tools in the safety improvement arsenal. These tools can be used to measure organizational conditions that lead to adverse events and patient harm, and for developing and evaluating safety improvement interventions in health care organizations. They provide a metric by which the implicit shared understandings about "the way we do things around here" can be made visible and available as input for change.

Health care organizations are only beginning to work with culture assessment tools and with the concept of safety culture itself. There is more to learn regarding creating and sustaining culture change in health care and the tools that might be used in these transformation efforts. Much remains to be discovered on how to use culture data in combination with other sources of information about safety improvement needs in different organizational contexts. Like other new safety improvement tools, there is room for further development on several fronts: accumulating evidence about the validity of these tools, learning how to initiate and sustain safety culture change, and discovering how to use culture data in combination with other sources of information about patient safety.

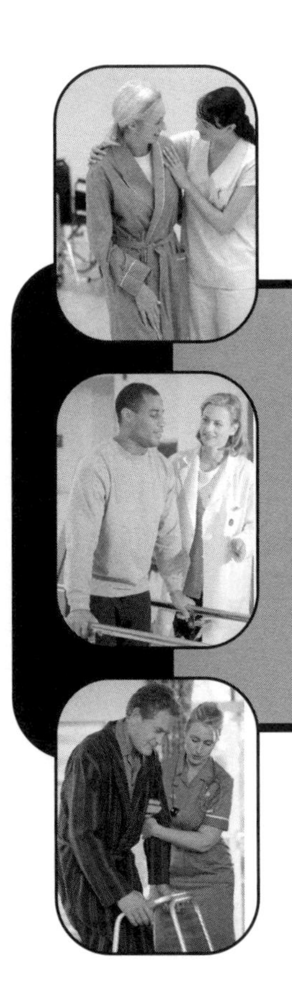

CHAPTER 1

Defining the Problem of Falls

Anna was an 85-year-old resident of a long term care facility. Generally quite lucid, Anna became disoriented following a change in her medications. Late one night, when she left her bed to use the bathroom, Anna fell and fractured her hip. The shock to her system was severe, and Anna died two days later. Anna's family filed a lawsuit, charging the facility with carelessness in not doing more to reduce the risk of Anna's fall.

How often does a fall like this occur? How would this fall be classified? What are the root causes of falls such as this? How does this fall apply to the reporting requirements of a sentinel event?

These are among the questions explored in this chapter and throughout this book. The stark reality is that despite great strides in reduction efforts over the last several decades, falls account for a significant portion of injuries among hospitalized patients, long term care residents, and home care recipients.[1, 2] The elderly are particularly susceptible. Approximately one third of adults over age 65 are reported to fall each year.[3] Those living in institutions fall three times that rate (1.5 falls per bed per year), with as many as 25% of institutional falls resulting in fracture, laceration, or need for hospital care.[4]

It is acknowledged that reducing falls among care recipients in any health care setting requires a multifaceted approach, and that the recognition, evaluation, and reduction of falls are significant challenges for all who are committed to providing a safe environment. Building, improving, and redesigning a comprehensive fall reduction program involves various stages of development.

In setting the groundwork for any implementation plans, this chapter looks at how falls are defined and classified, as well as the frequency of falls, the common causes of falls, and both the physical and financial costs associated with falls. It concludes with a review of the standards and requirements issued to accredited health care organizations by the Joint Commission.

Defining Falls

Falls continue to be defined and reported in different ways because no one definition has been universally accepted. Yet it is vitally important that each organization establish its own fall definition in order to accurately and consistently track and trend fall data. Definitions that have been recognized include the following:

- Patients or residents who experience an unplanned descent to the floor[5]
- An unintended event resulting in a person coming to rest on the ground/floor or other lower level (witnessed), or reportedly landing on the floor (unwitnessed) not due to any intentional movement or extrinsic force such as stroke, fainting, or seizure[6]
- An event that results in the patient or resident, or a body part of the patient or resident, coming to rest inadvertently on the ground or other surface lower than the patient or resident[7]
- An untoward event that results in the patient or resident coming to rest unintentionally on the ground or other lower surface

After the definition is crafted, it must be accepted by the organization's health care workers in order to be effectively and appropriately utilized in the completion of incident reports. One controversial element in a fall definition is whether to include a patient or resident assisted or lowered to the floor. When benchmarking against other organizations, the definition of inconsistencies needs to be noted to ensure that caution is used during analysis.

A historical way of reporting falls is by number of patients or residents per department. However, this method of reporting created inconsistencies for analysis of data such that there was no way of knowing if the increase was due to increased patient or resident census, increased admissions, or an increased number of incident reports.

To reduce the number of falls and improve overall safety, it is important that the starting point for all reporting and analysis begins with an organization's clear, consistent, and fully communicated definition of falls.

The Frequency of Falls

Falls are the leading cause of injury-related visits to emergency departments in the United States, the leading cause of trauma-related hospitalizations in the United States, and the primary etiology of accidental deaths in persons over the age of 65. The elderly, who represent 12% of the population, account for 75% of deaths from falls.[8] The number of falls increases progressively with age in both sexes and all racial and ethnic groups.[9] The injury rate for falls is highest among persons 85 years of age and older (for example, 171 deaths per 100,000 white men in this age group).[10] Approximately 9,500 deaths in older Americans are associated with falls each year.[11]

Falls are also a common cause of morbidity, occurring in all types of health care institutions' populations. National statistics published by the Centers for Disease Control and Prevention (CDC) refer to falls among older adults as a serious public health problem, primarily because falls result in more serious injury among this population. According to the CDC statistics for older adults, one in every three will sustain a fall each year.

The Joint Commission identified falls as one of the top five sentinel events for home care organizations in its December 2003 sentinel event report. Between 15% and 44.9% of community-dwelling elderly persons and up to 60% of nursing home residents fall each year; one half of these "fallers" have multiple episodes.[12]

In hospitals, patient falls consistently make up the largest single category of reported incidents. In U.S. nursing homes, approximately 1,800 fatal falls occur among residents each year,[13] with about 10% to 20% causing serious injuries. According to the CDC, these falls can result in decreased physical functioning, disability, and reduced quality of life. Loss of confidence and fear of falling can lead to further functional decline, depression, feelings of helplessness, and social isolation.

The CDC's *Falls in Nursing Homes Fact Sheet* reports the following:

- In 1997 1.5 million persons age 65 and older lived in nursing homes. If current rates continue, by 2030 this number will rise to about 3 million.
- Each year, a typical 100-bed nursing home reports 100 to 200 falls. Many others go unreported.
- As many as 75% of nursing home residents fall annually—twice the rate of seniors living in communities.
- Residents often experience multiple falls—2.6 falls per person per year on average.
- About 35% of fall injuries occur among nonambulatory residents.
- About 20% of all fall-related deaths among older adults occur among the 5% who live in nursing homes.

Falls occur more often in nursing homes because, generally, nursing home residents are frailer than seniors living in a community. Residents tend to be older, have more cognitive impairments, and have greater limitations in their activities of daily living. Residents also tend to have more chronic illnesses, be physically dependent, and have a higher prevalence of walking problems.[14]

Classifying Falls and Fall Risk

In developing the parameters of an accepted definition for falls, many organizations have chosen to classify falls based on environmental and physiologic factors in an effort to better understand its causes. Researcher Janice Morse suggests that falls be classified as accidental, unanticipated physiologic, or anticipated physiologic, as defined below:[15]

Accidental falls occur when care recipients fall unintentionally. For example, they may trip, slip, or fall because of a failure of equipment or by environmental factors such as spilled water or urine on the floor.

Unanticipated physiologic falls occur when the physical cause of the falls is not reflected in the care recipient's risk factor for falls. A fall in one of these cases is caused by physical conditions that cannot be predicted until the fall occurs. For example, the fall may be due to fainting, a seizure, or a pathological fracture of the hip.

Anticipated physiologic falls occur in care recipients whose score on risk assessment scales indicates that they are at risk of falling. According to the Morse Fall Scale, these care recipients have some of the following characteristics: a prior fall, weak or impaired gait, use of a walking aid, intravenous access, or impaired mental status.

According to Morse, approximately 14% of all falls in hospitals are accidental, another 8% are unanticipated physiologic falls, and 78% are anticipated physiologic falls.

It is generally accepted that falls are caused by multiple factors. Factors that place residents at risk for falls include a previous history of falls, cognitive impairment, impaired balance or mobility, musculoskeletal problems, chronic diseases, nutritional problems, and use of multiple medications.

Another popular classification method of falls is based on the assumption that a fall can result from a complex interaction of intrinsic and/or extrinsic risk factors. The summary list that follows is derived from many studies incorporating different methodologies, settings, samples, and overall quality. Individual risk factors may not be generalized across all settings, and may not be applicable to a particular organization.

Intrinsic risk factors are integral to the care recipient's system, many of which are associated with age-related changes:

- *Previous fall*—Studies have cited a history of falls as a significant factor associated with care recipients being more likely to fall again.
- *Reduced vision*—Vision affected by, for example, a decline in visual acuity, decreased night vision, altered depth perception, decline in peripheral vision, or glare intolerance
- *Unsteady gait*—Manner and style of walking
- *Musculoskeletal system*—Impact from factors such as muscle atrophy, calcification of tendons and ligaments, and increased curvature of the spine (osteoporosis) are associated with ability to maintain balance and proper posture.
- *Mental status*—Status affected by confusion, disorientation, inability to understand, and impaired memory
- *Acute illnesses*—Rapid onset of symptoms associated with seizures, stroke, orthostatic hypotension, and febrile conditions
- *Chronic illnesses*—Conditions such as arthritis, cataracts, glaucoma, dementia, diabetes and Parkinson's disease

Extrinsic risk factors are external to the system and relate to the physical environment:

- *Medications.* Those that affect the central nervous system, such as sedatives and tranquilizers, benzodiazepines, and the number of administered drugs
- *Bathtubs and toilets.* Equipment without support, such as grab bars
- *Design of furnishings.* Height of chairs and beds
- *Condition of ground surfaces.* Floor coverings with loose or thick-pile carpeting, sliding rugs, upended linoleum or tile flooring, highly polished or wet ground surfaces
- *Poor illumination conditions.* Intensity or glare issues
- *Type and condition of footwear.* Ill-fitting shoes or incompatible soles such as rubber crepe soles, which, though slip resistant, may stick to linoleum floor surfaces
- *Improper use of devices.* Bedside rails and mechanical restraining devices that may actually increase fall risk in some instances
- *Inadequate assistive devices.* Walkers, wheelchairs, and lifting devices[16]

Intrinsic Factors

As illustrated above, intrinsic factors involve characteristics that are inherent to each individual and are the result of changes related to aging, disease, or medication. It should be noted that Morse and others have suggested that this model does not necessarily categorize all falls and only partially directs approaches to interventions.

In his report, *The Changing Approach to Falls in the Elderly,*[17] Kenneth K. Steinweg, M.D., explains that simply maintaining a stable, upright position "involves a number of human systems and requires extensive sensory input, central integration, and musculoskeletal coordi-

SIDEBAR 1-1

Age-Related Factors Affecting Stability

Changes in postural control
- Decreased proprioception
- Slower righting reflexes
- Decreased muscle tone and strength
- Increased postural sway

Changes in gait
- Lower foot swing
- Slower gait

Declining visual abilities
- Depth perception
- Clarity
- Adaptation to the dark
- Color sensitivity
- Declining visual fields
- Visuospacial function
- Increased sensitivity to glare[18]

SIDEBAR 1-2

Pathologic Conditions Contributing to Falls in Elderly Care Recipients

- Arthritis
- Stroke
- Hip fractures
- Peripheral neuropathies
- Dementia
- Amputation
- Parkinson's syndrome
- Foot disorders and deformities

nation in a highly integrated manner." He also cites several age-related physiologic factors that contribute to instability and falls through their impact on these interrelated systems at multiple levels (*see* Sidebar 1-1, above). Many elderly persons experience gait changes related to aging. For men, the changes typically result in a decreased height of step. In women these changes tend to result in a narrow, waddling gait.

Vision also plays an extremely important role in balance. Steinweg's report suggests that acuity may decline as much as 80% by age 90, significantly impacting contrast sensitivity. This impairs an individual's ability to perceive object contrasts and spatial detail. In detecting objects in the environment, older persons require three times as much contrast as others. Their light-dark adaptation is slowed. There is more glare as a result of cataracts, and accommodation to changes in distance declines rapidly.[19]

Beyond the evolving physiologic changes of aging are the alterations in physiology caused by both acute and chronic conditions (*see* Sidebar 1-2, above). Compounding the changes of aging or even introducing new risk factors are conditions that affect sensory input, central processing, and musculoskeletal coordination. Conditions that affect the lower extremities are especially important.

Additionally, a number of age-related changes predispose an individual to orthostatic hypotension. Elderly persons are also susceptible to postprandial hypotension. According to Steinweg, as many as 16% of elderly care recipients might have had orthostatic hypotension, while patients or residents being treated for significant hypertension had rates of orthostatic hypotension almost twice as high. Finally, the simultaneous use of diuretics, anticholinergics, antihypertensives, and psychoactive medications also contribute to the propensity for orthostasis.

As the number of risk factors increases, the chance of a fall also increases.[20] However, Steinweg's research shows that risk can be minimized by modifying even a few contributing factors. Interventions such as improving vision, choosing proper footwear, and performing appropriate strengthening exercises can decrease the risks of falling.

Extrinsic Factors

Extrinsic factors also play important roles in falls and are often included in the "accident" category when causes of falls are analyzed. Homes of the elderly often contain many environmental hazards (*see* Sidebar 1-3, below).

While poor lighting compounds the visual changes associated with aging, the most commonly cited extrinsic cause of falls include loose rugs, slippery floors, and uneven door thresholds. Falls may also occur when bathroom fixtures and home furnishings are inappropriately low or high or without arm supports.

Approximately 10% of falls are associated with stairs. This may be related to a combination of inadequate handrails, poor vision, and weak lower extremity musculature. Reviewing these factors with elderly care recipients will aid in evaluating the safety of a home, as well as in eliciting the details of a fall.

SIDEBAR 1-3

Extrinsic Factors Related to Falls in the Elderly

- Poor lighting
- Slick or irregular floor surfaces
- Furnishings that are too low or too high
- Unsafe stairways
- Bathroom fixtures that are too low or too high or do not have arm supports
- Area rugs/throw rugs

Medication

Medication also plays a prominent role in the cause of falls. According to recent studies, between 20% and 30% of home care residents are at risk for potential medication errors. Medication errors occurring in the home result in harm 11% of the time, according to the U.S. Pharmacopeia's Safe Medication Use Expert Committee.[21,22] Of the harmful errors, 12% result in permanent harm, a life-threatening situation, or death.

Home care residents are vulnerable to medication errors for several reasons, according to the U.S. Pharmacopeia's Safe Medication Use Expert Committee. The majority of these residents are elderly. Of those, many are frail. They take several medications, which are often prescribed by more than one physician. Although some home care residents have multiple caregivers, some have none.

Consequently, home care organizations must be vigilant in monitoring medication errors and determining the causes when they occur to implement processes and programs to reduce the risk of reoccurrence.

Common Causes of Falls

Even older people who appear to be strong and well can fall. The normal changes of aging, such as poor eyesight or poor hearing, can make a person more likely to fall. Chapter 2 offers a more in-depth analysis of the root causes of care recipient falls and presents intervention strategies to help reduce such falls, but in defining falls it is important to note the factors that have been identified as common causes of falls in the elderly.

Falls and concomitant instability can be markers of poor health and declining function.[23] In older care recipients, a fall may be a nonspecific presenting sign of many acute illnesses, such as pneumonia, urinary tract infection, or myocardial infarction, or it may be the sign of acute exacerbation of a chronic disease.[24]

According to research from the American Academy of Family Physicians (AAFP), illnesses and physical conditions can impact a person's strength and balance, increasing his or her risk of falling. Environmental factors such as poor lighting or throw rugs in the home or in a health care setting can make a person more likely to trip or slip. Sidebar 1-4, below, offers some common causes of falls in the elderly.

The AAFP has also reported that the side effects of some medicines can upset a person's balance and contribute to a fall. Medications, especially psychoactive drugs such as sedatives and antianxiety drugs, can increase the risk of falls and fall-related injuries. Medicines for such issues as depression, sleep problems, and high blood pressure can cause a person to fall.

SIDEBAR 1-4

Common Causes of Falls in the Elderly*

- Accident, environmental hazard, fall from bed
- Gait disturbance, balance disorders or weakness, pain related to arthritis
- Vertigo
- Medications or alcohol
- Acute illness
- Confusion and cognitive impairment
- Postural hypotension
- Visual disorder
- Central nervous system disorder, syncope, drop attacks, epilepsy[25]

* *Listed in approximate order of occurrence*

Some medicines for diabetes and heart conditions can also make a person unsteady. People who take four or more medicines of these types may be more likely to fall. People who change their medicine within a two-week span are also more likely to fall because of interactions with their other medications. Table 1-1, page 21, looks at risk factors for injurious falls, as well as medications that may increase the likelihood of a fall.

According to the CDC, weakness and walking or gait problems are the most common causes of falls among nursing home residents, accounting for about 24% of the falls in nursing homes. The CDC also reported that environmental hazards account for 16% to 27% of nursing home falls. Such hazards include wet floors, poor lighting, lack of bed rails when they are indicated, clutter, incorrect bed height, and improperly maintained or fitted wheelchairs.

One researcher developed the mnemonic key in Sidebar 1-5, page 21, to spotlight the physical findings in the elderly who have fallen or are at risk of a fall.

Other causes include difficulty in transferring (for example, moving from the bed to a chair), poor foot care, poorly fitting shoes, and inappropriate or incorrect use of walking aids.[27] In recent years, some experts have contended that the use of restraints can actually contribute to fall-related injuries and deaths because limiting the care recipient's freedom of movement leads to muscle weakness and reduces physical function.[28]

The Physical Costs of Falls

The morbidity, mortality, and financial burdens attributed to falls in hospitals and other health care settings are among the most serious risk-management issues facing the health care industry. For the patient or resident, consequences include, but are not limited to, fracture, soft

SIDEBAR 1-5

I Hate Falling: A Mnemonic for Key Physical Findings in the Elderly Person Who Falls or Nearly Falls

I	Inflammation of joints (or joint deformity)
H	Hypotension (orthostatic blood pressure changes)
A	Auditory and visual abnormalities
T	Tremor (Parkinson's disease or other causes of tremor)
E	Equilibrium (balance) problem
F	Foot problems
A	Arrhythmia, heart block, or valvular disease
L	Leg-length discrepancy
L	Lack of conditioning (generalized weakness)
I	Illness
N	Nutrition (poor weight loss)
G	Gait disturbance[26]

tissue or head injury, fear of falling, anxiety, and depression.

As mentioned previously, falls are the leading cause of injury or death among people age 65 and older. In 1997 (the most recent data available) about 9,000 people over the age of 65 died from fall-related injuries. Elderly persons who survive a fall experience significant morbidity. Hospital stays are almost twice as long in the elderly who are hospitalized after a fall than in the elderly who are admitted for another reason.[29] Compared with elderly persons who do not fall, those who fall experience greater functional decline in activities of daily living and in physical and social activities,[30] and they are at greater risk for subsequent institutionalization.[31]

Major injuries, including head trauma, soft tissue injuries, fractures, and dislocations, occur in 5% to 15% of falls in any given year. Fractures account for 75% of serious injuries, with hip fractures occurring in 1% to 2% of falls.[32] Hip fracture is the leading fall-related injury that results in hospitalization, with these hospital stays being significantly prolonged and costly.[33] More than 90% of hip fractures are associated with falls, and most of these fractures occur in persons more than 70 years of age.[34]

According to the CDC, the following is true in the United States:

- Of all fractures, hip fractures cause the greatest number of deaths and lead to the most severe health problems. There were approximately 340,000 hospital admissions for hip fractures in 1996 (the most recent data available). This incidence is expected to double by the middle of the twenty-first century.
- Falls account for 87% of all fractures for people age 65 or older. Falls are also the second leading cause of spinal cord and brain injury among older adults.
- Older adults are hospitalized for fall-related injuries five times more often than they are for injuries from other causes.
- Of those who fall, 20% to 30% suffer moderate to severe injuries that reduce mobility and independence, and increase the risk of premature death.
- Among seniors, falls are the underlying cause of a large proportion of fatal traumatic brain injuries (TBI). From 1989 to 1998, the fall-

TABLE 1-1

Risk Factors for Injurious Falls and Medications

Risk factors for injurious falls

- Previous falls
- Cognitive impairment
- Impaired balance, gait, strength
- Neurologic disease (for example, stroke, Parkinson's disease)
- Musculoskeletal disease (for example, arthritis, joint replacement, deformity, foot problems, sensory impairment)
- Chronic disease (for example, osteoporosis, cardiovascular disease, lung disease, diabetes)
- Impaired mobility
- Problems with nutrition
- Medications
- Number of prescription medications (for example, sedatives, antidepressants, neuroleptics, antihypertensive medications, diuretics); greater than four associated with increased risk
- Addition of risk factors in someone already at risk (for example, introduction of new medications likely to affect balance, flare of chronic disease)

Medications that may predispose individuals to fall

- Antiarrhythmics
- Antidepressants
- Antihypertensives
- Diuretics
- Hypoglycemics
- Laxatives
- Neuroleptics
- Nonsteroidal anti-inflammatory agents
- Psychotropics
- Sedatives/hypnotics
- Vasodilators

induced TBI death rate among people age 80 and older increased 60%.

- The risk of falling increases exponentially with age.
- Older adults who have fallen previously, or who stumble frequently, are two to three times more likely to fall within the next year.
- For people age 65 and older, two thirds to one half of falls occur in or around the home.

The Financial Costs of Falls

On the financial end, fall-related injuries recently accounted for 6% of all medical expenditures for people age 65 and older in the United States. In the last several years, the CDC has made an effort to calculate cost estimates for fall-related injuries. These calculations focused on direct costs, which include out-of-pocket expenses and charges paid by insurance companies for the treatment of fall-related injuries. These include costs and fees associated with hospital and nursing home care, physician and other professional services, rehabilitation, community-based services, the use of medical equipment, prescription drugs, local rehabilitation, home modifications, and insurance administration. Direct costs do not, however, account for the long-term consequences of these injuries, such as disability, decreased productivity, or reduced quality of life.

The total cost of all fall injuries for people age 65 or older in 1994 was $20.2 billion. By 2020 the cost of fall injuries is expected to reach $32.4 billion, before adjusting for inflation. A recent study of people age 72 and older found that the average health care cost of a fall injury was $19,440 (including hospital, nursing home, emergency room, and home health care, but not physician services).

Focusing on fall-related fractures, the CDC reports the following:

- The most common fall-related injuries are osteoporotic fractures. These are fractures of the hip, spine, or forearm.
- In the United States in 1986, the direct medical costs for osteoporotic fractures were $5.15 billion. By 1989 these costs exceeded $6 billion.
- A study published in 1994 estimated that total direct medical costs for osteoporotic fractures among postmenopausal women in the next 10 years would be more than $45.2 billion.
- Of all fall-related fractures, hip fractures are the most serious and lead to the greatest number of health problems and deaths.
- In the United States, hospitalization accounts for 44% of direct health care costs for hip fracture care recipients. In 1991 Medicare costs for this injury were estimated to be $2.9 billion.
- Hospital admissions for hip fractures among people over age 65 have steadily increased, from 230,000 admissions in 1988 to 338,000 admissions in 1999. The number of hip fractures is expected to exceed 500,000 per year by 2040.

The CDC report concludes, "Assuming 5% inflation and the growing number of hip fractures, the total annual cost of these injuries is projected to reach $240 billion by the year 2040."

The following scenario provides a look at how a care recipient fall can result in tragic human consequences, a sentinel event, and possibly costly litigation.

A 75- year-old male with advanced pancreatic cancer was admitted to a hospice. The admission assessment determined he was at greater risk of a fall because of his history (three falls within the last six weeks) and because of his periodic mental confusion and weakened condition. Fall precautions were initiated that included positioning the bed in a low position and the use of a bed alarm.

During the first two days it was observed that he made at least two attempts to get out of bed; however, each time a staff member was able to intervene. On the third day at 3:00 A.M., the nursing assistant on rounds noticed the care recipient sitting on the floor next to his bed. Upon investigation it was discovered that the bed alarm had been disconnected by the 3:00 P.M. to 11:00 P.M. shift during a linen change and not reconnected.

The care recipient suffered a fractured femur and died within 48 hours of the incident. The care recipient's daughter filed a liability claim against the hospice alleging that the organization was negligent in failing to provide a safe environment for her father, resulting in an injury that contributed to his death. The demand for damages was $250,000.

Joint Commission Requirements Related to Falls

Fatal falls rank high on the list of sentinel events tracked by the Joint Commission. Approximately 4.9% of the sentinel events reviewed by the Joint Commission through the end of 2004 were due to falls. A *sentinel event* is an unexpected occurrence involving death or serious physical or psychological injury, or the risk thereof. The phrase *or the risk thereof* includes any process variation for which a recurrence would carry a significant chance of a serious adverse outcome. Such events are called *sentinel* because they signal the need for immediate investigation and response.

When the care recipients and/or their families seek legal recourse to injuries caused by a sentinel event, the cases are often challenging, complex, and expensive. The elements of a basic malpractice action apply to an analysis of the liability issues involved with a fall. The standard of care is "what a reasonable person with the same degree of experience and expertise would do in the same or similar circumstances."[35] The organization, therefore, must be concerned with the specific facts of the case and whether a reasonable standard of care was followed. If the organization's policies and procedures regarding sentinel events are followed, data collection and analysis can determine whether a reasonable standard of care was breached.

Each Joint Commission accreditation manual contains standards in the Improving Organization Performance (PI) chapter that relate specifically to the management of sentinel events. These standards are PI.1.10, PI.2.20, PI.2.30, and PI.3.10. Standard PI.2.30 requires each accredited organization to define *sentinel event* for its own purposes in establishing mechanisms to identify, report, and manage these events. Although this definition must be consistent with the general definition of sentinel events as published by the Joint Commission, accredited organizations have some latitude in setting more specific parameters to define *unexpected, serious,* and *the risk thereof.* At a minimum, an organization's definition must include those events that are subject to review under the Sentinel Event Policy as defined in the Joint Commission's accreditation manuals.

Accredited organizations are expected to identify and respond appropriately to all sentinel events occurring in the organization or associated with services that the organization provides, or provides for. Appropriate response includes conducting a timely, thorough, and credible root cause analysis; developing an action plan designed to implement improvements to reduce risk; implementing the improvements; and monitoring the effectiveness of those improvements.

These and other sentinel event requirements and guidelines are detailed in the Joint Commission's accreditation manuals. As described in these manuals, the Joint Commission collects and analyzes data from the review of sentinel events, root cause analyses, action plans, and follow-up activities. These data and information form the content of the Joint Commission's Sentinel Event Database. The Joint Commission is committed to developing and maintaining this Sentinel Event Database in a fashion that protects the confidentiality of the organization, the caregiver, and the care recipient. Included in this database are the following three major categories of data elements:

1. Sentinel event data
2. Root cause data
3. Risk reduction data

The Sentinel Event Database is also a major component of the evidence base for the National Patient Safety Goals. Accredited organizations are evaluated for continuous compliance with the specific requirements associated with the National Patient Safety Goals.

The Joint Commission's Sentinel Event

Advisory Group has recommended National Patient Safety Goals and associated requirements for 2006. The 2006 Goals are program specific and apply to ambulatory care, office-based surgery, assisted living, behavioral health care, critical access hospitals, disease-specific care, home care, hospitals, laboratories, long term care, integrated delivery systems, managed care organizations, and preferred provider organizations. The Joint Commission made the National Patient Safety Goals program specific to increase the relevance of the Goals and requirements to the individuals served in each program.

Two Goals deal specifically with the issue of falls. As described in Figure 1-1, Goal 8 addresses the accuracy of medications and treatments across the care continuum. The elderly who have had two or more falls use a significantly higher number of sedatives and hypnotics, analgesics, and cardiovascular agents than those who have not fallen or have fallen

FIGURE 1-1

Joint Commission National Patient Safety Goal 8

Goal 8: Accurately and completely reconcile medications across the continuum of care.
Requirement 8A: Implement a process for obtaining and documenting a complete list of the patient's/resident's current medications upon the patient's/resident's admission to the organization and with the involvement of the patient/resident (applicable to assisted living, critical access hospitals, home care, hospitals, long term care). This process includes a comparison of the medications the organization provides to those on the list (applicable to assisted living, critical access hospitals, hospitals, long term care).

Requirement 8B: A complete list of the patient's/resident's medication is communicated to the next provider of service when it refers or transfers a patient/resident to another setting, service, practitioner, or level of care within or outside the organization (applicable to assisted living, critical access hospitals, home care, hospitals, long term care).

Medication management encompasses the system and processes that an organization uses to provide medication to a care recipient throughout the continuum of care. There is a high risk for medication error or adverse drug event during handoffs in the continuum of care. Ensuring accuracy in the list of the care recipient's current medications at each instance of care is essential to providing safe care and reducing the risk of falls.

Few organizations have standard processes in place to reconcile medications when the care recipient enters the organization, or transfers through or out of the organization. A majority of medication errors occur at the initial points of contact in which a caregiver is admitting or transferring the care recipient to another floor in the hospital or to another health care organization. For example, the medication list can change significantly between the time the individual is discharged from the organization and reenters the organization. During that time, the regular or on-call physician could have changed the medications, or the medications could have been customized because of side effects or cost considerations. Therefore, the historical record that the organization uses may not always be accurate because the medications can change at any point. As a result, the organization must use many different resources, such as the historical record, an interview with the patient or resident and family, or a discussion with the care recipient's regular pharmacist or physician, to gain an accurate list of medications taken.

once. *Polypharmacy,* when five or more different drugs are prescribed concurrently, is also associated with falls.[36] The Goal also includes requirements that establish, upon admission, the involvement of the care recipient and previous care settings in obtaining comprehensive medication and treatment information.

Assisted living facilities, critical access hospitals, home care organizations, hospitals, and long term care facilities should assess and periodically reassess each care recipient's risk for falling, including the potential risk associated with the medication regimen. These organizations should also address any identified risks. Moreover, critical access hospitals, home care organizations, hospitals, and long term care organizations are required to implement a program of risk reduction—and evaluate the effectiveness of that program. This risk reduction program should include risk reduction strategies, staff in-services, involvement of care recipients/families in education, and evaluation of environment of care issues.

As described in Figure 1-2, Goal 9 of the National Patient Safety Goals addresses the issue of fall reduction measures and concludes that organizations that regularly assess each patient's or resident's risk for falling—and take action to reduce the likelihood of falls from happening—will succeed in reducing not just injuries, but also fatalities that result from falls.

All accredited organizations that provide care relevant to these Goals and requirements will be expected to comply with them. Compliance with all National Patient Safety Goals and requirements that are relevant to an organization's services will be evaluated for continuous compliance throughout the accreditation cycle through on-site surveys, Periodic Performance Review (PPR) for programs where PPR is applicable, and Evidence of Standards Compliance.

Surveyors will look for evidence of consistent implementation of the requirements. Regardless of when a survey is conducted during the year, scoring will be based on an expectation of continued compliance since January 1, 2005. Less than 100% compliance will result in a requirement for improvement.

This chapter has discussed the definitions of care recipient falls, the significance of fall problems, and the importance of systematic compliance in responding to falls. The following chapter discusses the root causes of falls. In presenting sentinel event examples for many of the root causes, the chapter also introduces intervention strategies designed to help shape a reduction approach to such causes.

FIGURE 1-2

Joint Commission National Patient Safety Goal 9

Goal 9: Reduce the risk of patient/resident harm resulting from falls.
Requirement 9B: Implement a fall reduction program and evaluate the effectiveness of the program.

Joint Commission Requirement
An organization should regularly assess each patient's/resident's risk for falling and take action to reduce the risk of falls. This includes risk factors such as previous history of falls, cognitive impairment, impaired balance or mobility, musculoskeletal problems, chronic diseases, nutritional problems, and use of multiple medications. This program should include risk reduction strategies, in-services, involvement of residents/families in education, and evaluation of environment of care issues. The program should also include development and implementation of transfer protocols (for example, bed-to-chair) when relevant.

References

1. Rubenstein L., Josephson K., Robbins A.: Falls in the nursing home. *Ann Intern Med* 121:442–451, 1994.
2. Doweiko D.: Prevention program cut patient falls by 10%. *Hosp Case Manag* 38:43–44, 2000.
3. Rubenstein L., Powers C., MacLean C.: Quality indicators for the management and prevention of falls and mobility problems in vulnerable elders (ACOVE). *Ann Intern Med* 135 (pt. 2):686–693, 2001.
4. Hoskin A.: Fatal falls: Trends and characteristics. *Stat Bull Metrop Life Found* 79:10–15, 1998.
5. Morris E.V., Isaacs B.: The prevention of falls in a geriatric hospital. *Age Ageing* 9:181–185, Mar. 1980.
6. Patient Safety Steering Committee: [Chapter on Falls Prevention Initiative]. In *Building the Foundations for Patient Safety.* Florida Hospital Association, 2001.
7. Kellogg International Work Group on the Prevention of Falls by the Elderly: The prevention of falls in later life. *Dan Med Bull* 34:1–24, Apr. 1987.
8. Greenhouse A.H.: Falls among the elderly. In Albert M.L., Knoefel J.E. (eds.): *Clinical Neurology of Aging,* 2nd ed. New York: Oxford University Press, 1994, pp. 611–626.
9. Tibbits G.M.: Patients who fall: How to predict and prevent injuries. *BMC Geriatr* 51:24–28, 31, 1996.
10. Sattin R.W.: Falls among older persons: A public health perspective. *Annu Rev Public Health* 13:489–508, 1992.
11. Capezuti E.: Falls. In Lavizzo-Mourey R.J., Forciea M.A. (eds.): *Geriatric Secrets.* Philadelphia: Hanley & Belfus, 1996, pp. 110–115.
12. Hirsch C.H., et al.: The natural history of functional morbidity in hospitalized older patients. *J Am Geriatr Soc* 38:1296–1303, 1990.
13. Rubenstein L.Z., et al.: Falls and instability in the elderly. *J Am Geriatr Soc* 36:266–278, 1988.
14. Bedsine R.W., Rubenstein L.Z., Snyder L. (eds): *Medical Care of the Nursing Home Resident.* Philadelphia: American College of Physicians, 1996.
15. Morse, J.M.: Enhancing the safety of hospitalization by reducing patient falls. *Am J Infect Control* 30:376–380, Jun. 2002.
16. Tideiksaar R.: *Falls in Older People: Prevention and Management,* 3rd ed. Baltimore: Health Professions Press, 2002.
17. Steinweg K.K.: The changing approach to falls in the elderly. *Am Fam Physician,* 56:1–11, Jul. 1997.
18. Instability and falls. In Kane R.L., Ouslander J.G., Abrass I.B. (eds.): *Essentials of Clinical Geriatrics,* 3rd ed. New York: McGraw-Hill, 1994, p. 200.
19. Tideiksaar R.: *Falling in Old Age: Prevention and Management,* 2rd ed. New York: Springer Publishing, 1997, pp. 6–7.
20. Robbins A.S., et al.: Predictors of falls among elderly people; Results of two population-based studies. *Arch Intern Med* 149:1628–1633, 1989.
21. Meredith, S.: Possible medication errors in home healthcare patients. *JAGS* 49:719–724, Jun., 2001.
22. Zahn C.: Potentially inappropriate medication use in the community-dwelling elderly: Findings from the 1996 medical expenditure panel survey. *JAMA* 286:2823–2829, 2001.
23. Tinetti M.E., et al.: Shared risk factors for falls, incontinence, and functional dependence: Unifying the approach to geriatric syndromes. *JAMA* 273:1348–1353, 1995.
24. Rabin D.W.: Falls and gait disorders. In Abrams W.B., Beers M.H., Berkow R. (eds.): *The Merck Manual of Geriatrics,* 2nd ed. Rahway, NJ: Merck Sharp & Dohme Research Laboratories, 1995, pp. 65–78.
25. Fuller G.F.: Falls in the elderly. American Academy of Family Physicians. Apr. 1, 2000. http://www.aafp.org/afp/20000401/2159.html (accessed Feb. 4, 2005).
26. Sloan J.P.: Mobility failure. In *Protocols in Primary Care Geriatrics.* New York: Springer, 1997, pp. 33–38.
27. Rubenstein L.Z.: Falls. In Yoshikawa T.T., Cobbs E.L., Brummel-Smith K. (eds.): *Ambulatory Geriatric Care.* St. Louis: Mosby, 1993, pp. 296–304.
28. Rubenstein L.Z.: Preventing falls in the nursing home. *JAMA* 278:595–596, Jul. 1997.
29. Dunn J.E., et al.: Mortality, disability, and falls in older persons: The role of underlying disease and disability. *Am J Public Health* 82:395–400, 1992.
30. Kiel D.P., et al.: Health care utilization and functional status in the aged following a fall. *Med Care* 29:221–228, 1991.

31. Tinetti M.E., Liu W.L., Claus E.B.: Predictors and prognosis of inability to get up after falls among elderly persons. *JAMA* 269:65–70, 1993.
32. King M.B., Tinetti M.E.: A multifactorial approach to reducing injurious falls. *Clin Geriatr Med* 12:745–759, 1996.
33. Mahoney J.E.: Immobility and falls. *Clin Geriatr Med* 14:699–726, 1998.
34. Rubenstein L.Z., Powers C.M., MacLean C.H.: Quality indicators for the management and prevention of falls and mobility problems in vulnerable elders (ACOVE). *Ann Intern Med* 135(pt. 2):686–693, 2001.
35. Willey E., Youngberg B.: Education as a valuable risk management resource. In Youngberg B. (ed.): *The Risk Manager's Desk Reference*. Gaithersburg, MD:Aspen Publishers, Inc. 1994, p. 72.
36. Von Renteln-Kruse W.: Falls in the elderly and drugs. *Z Gerontol Geriatr* 30:276–280, 1997.

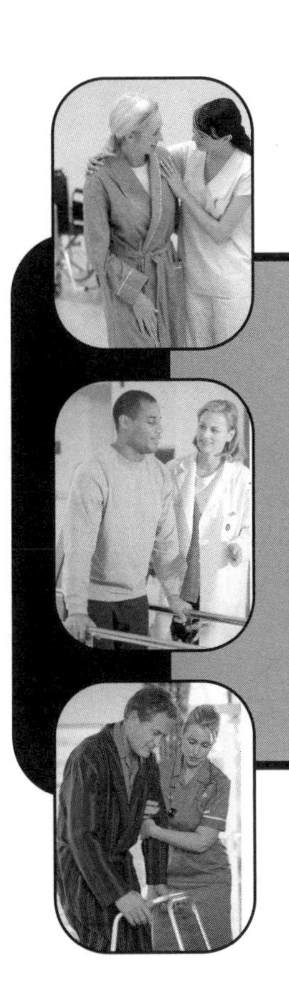

CHAPTER 2

Strategies for Addressing the Root Causes of Falls

A large health care organization is experiencing the effects of flu season. The census is increasing, as is the number of staff out ill. The long term care unit needs one full-time registered nurse in addition to a licensed practical nurse, a nurse manager, and three nursing assistants. When the nurse covering the 7:00 A.M. to 3:00 P.M. shift calls in ill, the nurse manager does not request a replacement registered nurse, and the nurse manager offers to assist on the unit. When the nurse manager is called into meetings at 10:00 A.M., she is not able to return to the unit, leaving the licensed practical nurse to oversee the unit. During lunch, when two of the three nursing assistants are taking a lunch break, three care recipients fall while attempting to get to the bathroom without assistance. All three individuals state that their request for assistance via the call light had not been met for a long time, so they attempted to make the walk unassisted due to their urgent need to use the bathroom. Fortunately, none were severely injured.

How did the lack of appropriate staff levels contribute to these falls? What role did staff communication play? What impact would staff training have had? Was the organization's environment of care a factor in this fall? Was the organization's care planning process effective in this incident?

One thing is particularly clear in the above: Maintaining adequate staffing levels is a key area of concern in reducing falls. Without adequate staffing, care recipients receive less assistance when needed, and caregivers receive less training and less supervision. These factors have a significant impact on both the number and severity of falls.

The example above is one of many explored in this chapter, and the questions it poses are among the many this chapter will attempt to answer. Beginning with an in-depth look at the root causes of care recipient falls and continuing with intervention strategies that can contribute to reducing falls, the pages ahead offer an overview of the situational outcomes that can result from a comprehensive fall-related injury reduction program.

Tracking the Root Causes of Falls

In its tracking of care recipient falls between 1995 and 2004, the Joint Commission review of sentinel events indicates that organizations reporting fatal falls identified several root causes for falls, which include the following:

- Staff issues such as inadequate caregiver communication, incomplete orientation and training of new staff, inadequate supervision of caregivers in training, and inadequate staffing levels
- Incomplete assessment or reassessment
- Environmental issues such as unsafe window design, door locks, or nursing stations, or malfunction or misuse of equipment
- Incomplete care planning, and unavailable or delayed care provision
- Inadequate organizational culture

Figure 2-1 provides a percentage breakdown of the root causes reported to the Joint Commission's latest sentinel event tracking efforts.

All sentinel events due to falls, according to the Joint Commission Sentinel Event Database, occurred in 24-hour care settings. Half of the falls involved individuals over the age of 80. A significant proportion of individuals who fell had an altered mental status due to acute or chronic illness (mental or physical). A history of

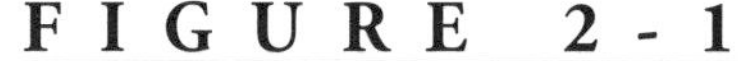

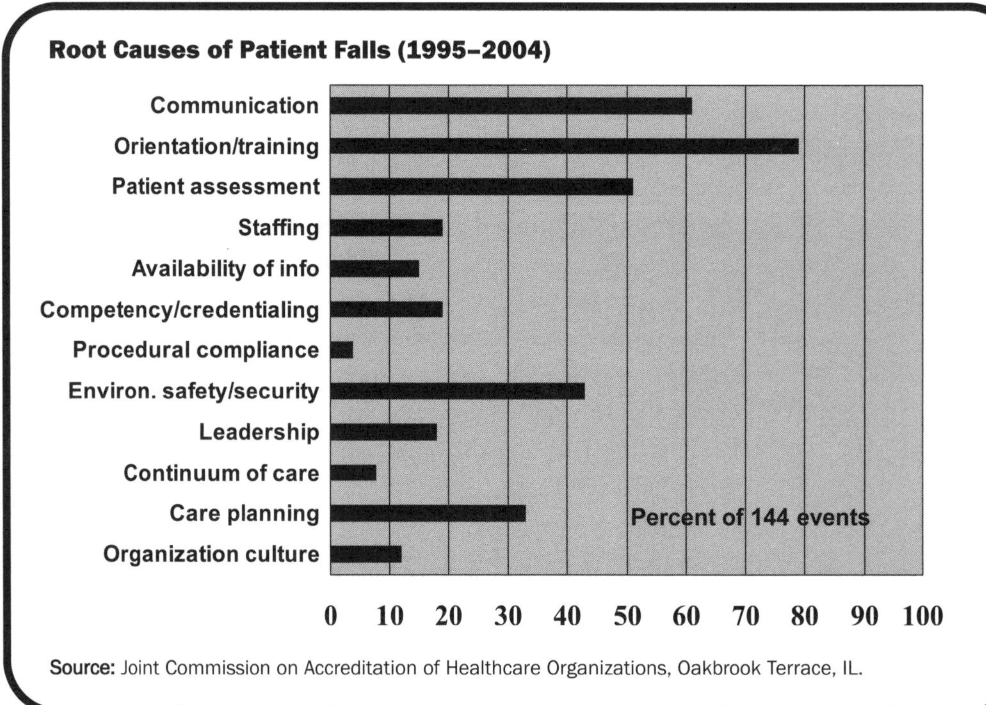

Source: Joint Commission on Accreditation of Healthcare Organizations, Oakbrook Terrace, IL.

prior falls, use of sedation, use of anticoagulant therapy, recent change of environment, and urinary urgency were frequently associated risk factors either for the fall or the resulting serious injury from the fall. Most of the falls occurred at night, on weekends, and on holidays—traditionally times of lower staffing levels.

Staff Communication, Orientation, and Training

The Joint Commission found that communication issues among caregivers, staff orientation and/or training, and care recipient assessment were the leading root causes of patient or resident falls. Of the 144 events reported to the Joint Commission during 2004, a total of 35 falls indicated a significant increase from 2003. These included failure to obtain adequate information related to fall history, failure to communicate information to staff during nursing report or shift change, and failure to document changes in conditions in the medical record.

A lack of information can inhibit the important process of developing and implementing an individualized care plan for those at risk of falling. If the changes in a care recipient's condition are not clearly and consistently communicated to other staff members, opportunities to make necessary risk-reduction adjustments to that individual's care plan may be missed. The ongoing observation of a care recipient is also more likely to be deficient, especially during shift changes, without a coordinated system of both written and verbal communication among staff.

"When you're dealing with an elderly, frail, or cognitively impaired population, falls are more likely to happen when staff members haven't been oriented to meet the residents' needs," says Marianna Kern Grachek, executive director of long term care and assisted living accreditation at the Joint Commission. "Ongoing communication must be maintained about the needs of the residents. As staff members come on duty, they should be made aware of the specific and changing needs of the patients/residents who are assigned to their care."

Problems arise when staff members must cover for others. For example, when a staff member goes on a work break, another staff member may need to assume responsibility for a resident but may not have been briefed on the resident's specific care needs. In addition, when the mobility and/or cognitive functioning of a resident changes, that information should be relayed in an ongoing manner and at shift change. "When there is a competing priority, staff members may be hurried and may not have an opportunity to share resident-specific information. As a result, they will not know the changing care needs of residents in their care," states Grachek. In shift reports, staff members need to be made aware of the residents' ability to manage their physical environment. "Staff members may need to modify the environment to accommodate the resident's limitations," says Grachek.

Care Recipient Assessment

Observation is critical to the assessment and reassessment of a care recipient. An initial assessment or follow-up assessment that fails to identify such risk factors as an individual's overall cognitive level, muscle strength, pain, toileting urgency and frequency, and ability to perform activities of daily living can lead to invalid conclusions about the individual's status and, therefore, increase that individual's risk of falling. Inadequate assessments not only increase the likelihood of staff implementing inadequate intervention strategies, but limit staff's ability to measure the desired impact of such interventions.

Physical Environment

Spills, hallway clutter, and slippery floors are among the environmental factors that can contribute to care recipient falls. If a wheelchair, walker, cane, or other equipment used by a care recipient are not in proper condition, they can also cause a fall. Falls can also occur when an organization's devices—such as bed exit alarms, chair exit alarms, and voice alarms—are not functioning properly. The risk of falls from these environment of care issues are compounded when staff are not fully trained and empowered to take action to address unsafe conditions. When staff fail to caution care recipients about such risks, another opportunity to reduce the risk of a fall is missed.

Care Planning

A care planning process that does not involve a multifactor, interdisciplinary approach can result in risk factors that go unrecognized. If a nursing care plan, which is generally the first step in this process, is not followed by an assessment of additional disciplines—such as medical, pharmacy, and physical/occupational therapy—a care recipient's care plan is potentially incomplete. For example, undocumented medication allergies place an individual at increased risk of adverse drug reactions and increased risk of falls. This interdisciplinary process relies on the strength of the team's communication process. In developing a successful care plan for individuals taking medications that increase the risk of falls, for example, a pharmacist must effectively educate and alert nurses and other staff about symptoms to look for.

Organizational Culture

As mentioned previously, if an institution's organizational culture is one in which acknowledgement of error or expressions of concern are not encouraged, then the greater possibilities of learning from experience are substantially limited. Without a sense of openness and, perhaps, vigilance in monitoring issues of safety, organizations help create an atmosphere in which inadequate care is inevitable. At the very core of any effort to improve safety and reduce the risk of falls is an environment that supports the open exchange of any and all relevant information that might reduce errors and mitigate the impact of errors that occur.[1]

Root Cause Cases and Intervention Strategies

Although the sentinel event scenarios below are addressed with corresponding intervention strategies, it is important to note that all of the suggested interventions are interrelated and combined with other measures to help define a multifactorial, interdisciplinary approach to fall reduction. Maintaining adequate staffing levels, for example, is essential to any and all designs toward reducing the risk of falls. The same can be said of improving staff orientation and training regarding fall risk assessment processes and orienting the entire staff about the formal fall reduction protocols that are in place. All strategies that are designed to reduce the risks of care recipient falls must be measured to fit each individual organization and its unique variables of risk.

Root Cause Example: Inadequate Caregiver Communication

Two days after a surgical procedure, a hospitalized man begins to experience increased weakness, unsteady balance, and forgetfulness. Nursing staff on the 3:00 P.M. to 11:00 P.M. shift reassess the patient and revise the care plan. They do not verbally communicate this information to staff on the following shift; the assigned nurse leaves before changing the documentation on the plan of care. Because the 11:00 P.M. to 7:00 A.M. shift does not have the benefit of this information, a nurse helps the man into a chair for breakfast and leaves him unattended. When the breakfast tray is brought into the room an hour later, the man is found sitting on the bathroom floor bleeding from a large head wound.

STRATEGY

Communicate and Coordinate

- Ensure continual observation of the individual.
- Ensure that care is provided in a coordinated manner.
- Communicate changes in condition and behaviors, especially during shift changes.
- Reassess and revise the care recipient's care plan.

Communication and transfer of information between and among health care professionals are essential to reducing fall risk. In the previous example, the incident could have been avoided if the man had not been left unattended for such a long time. Poor communication hindered the information flow from the evening shift to the night shift.

Coordinated communication can help staff revise care plans appropriately and implement proactive fall risk reduction strategies. Thorough communication among nursing staff and other team members helps to ensure that care is provided in a coordinated manner. By regular observation, staff can identify changes in condition, or behavior indicating problems or the need for care plan revision.

Communication during shift changes or setting transfers is particularly critical. For example, the night nurse must inform a nurse on the day shift in a long term care setting that an individual receiving pain medication complained of dizziness. Ideally, communication should be both written and verbal. Staff must ensure thorough documentation in the clinical record of the care recipient's response to care and services.

Nurses must communicate to all caregivers information concerning changes experienced by the care recipient. This must occur among all levels and all disciplines of staff, including administrative and environment care staff.

Documentation in the clinical record is essential and should be enhanced by a verbal report whenever possible. Nurses can tape-record change-of-shift reports for the next shift staff. Summarized 24-hour sheets or computerized report sheets that list significant changes in condition, as well as admissions and discharges, are a helpful communication tool. These can be checked by the shift supervisor when making unit rounds and delivered to the nursing supervisor's office at the end of each 24-hour period. Staff must make changes to the plan of care as soon as the need and approaches have been established. Individuals at risk of falling can be identified in care plan documents by a colored dot or other measure. To alert staff of fall risk, the colored dot can be placed over the head of the bed, on the chart, and at the entrance to the individual's room if regulations permit. As always, be sensitive to the care recipient's right to privacy and confidentiality of health care information.

Root Cause Example: Inadequate Staff Orientation and Training

Due to staff illness, a nurse normally working in the emergency area is assigned to the day surgery unit. The nurse informs his supervisor that he has not worked in the day surgery area for more than two years and does not feel prepared or competent to do so. His supervisor states that it is his turn to go and reminds him that he passed a written test of cross-department tasks last year and, therefore, is competent.

Unfamiliar with discharge criteria and assessing day surgery patients, the nurse discharges a man too early. Without assistance, the individual is allowed to get up and begin dressing to return home. The moment the nurse leaves the room, the man's already low blood pressure drops even lower and he falls to the floor, breaking a leg. The nurse returns and finds the man on the floor breathing shallowly. He quickly calls for and receives assistance to move the man back onto a stretcher, and reassesses and treats his condition.

STRATEGY

Trained and Ready

- All caregivers must be competent in addressing age-specific needs of care recipients and be trained to identify cognitive impairments, gait instability, or other conditions that place individuals at risk for falls.
- If an organization has a fall reduction program, all staff must be competent in program elements before providing care to individuals who are at risk of falling.

- *Understand the physiology of falls.* Staff must be well versed in the physiology of falls. As described by Russell Massaro, M.D., executive vice president for Joint Commission accreditation operations, "A fall is an assault on the normal physiology that keeps humans upright. Staying upright or walking are beautifully complex processes, integrating functions of the eyes, ears, sense of touch, neuromuscular system, nervous system, and cognitive abilities. These functions work together to create a dance in which walking is actually controlled falling. Every step a person takes is the beginning of a fall because gravity always wants us to fall."[2] Now consider a person who has abnormalities of the feet, like bunions or flat feet. Or perhaps the person wears bifocals, or takes medications for hypertension or depression. This person is at increased risk of falling. "A fall is usually the result of the confluence of effects of multiple minor challenges to the delicate balance that keeps us upright," states Massaro. Singular answers do not assist assessment or reduction efforts. Staff must understand the full realm of the challenge.
- *Know fall risk factors.* Staff must be knowledgeable about fall risk factors. Studies that correlate specific disease states and other factors, such as medications with increased fall risk, abound in health care literature. Staff should be familiar with identified fall risk factors, such as the knowledge that adults taking more than three or four medications—*polypharmacy*—are at risk of recurrent falls.
- *Know who is at risk for falling and implement the organization's fall reduction program.* Thorough assessment and use of successful intervention techniques are critical in identifying those at risk of falling and implementing the organization's fall reduction program. Educating the family or significant others about safety strategies can help reduce the risk of falls in the facility and after the individual is discharged. Staff must be well versed in effective education techniques. In addition, knowledge of how to effectively communicate fall risk, fall reduction strategies, and change in care recipients' conditions are critical to fall reduction.
- *Inform the supervisor of unsafe staffing situations.* As advocates for the individuals in their care, all staff members should communicate their concern about unsafe staffing situa-

tions. Notification of a supervisor and documentation through channels established by the organization are appropriate.

Although looking at the basic causes and reduction strategies for care recipient falls is integral to any fall reduction program, the process of establishing a comprehensive program involves much more than connecting causes to cures.

Root Cause Examples: Inadequate Assessment and Reassessment

Inadequate Time for Assessment

A man scheduled for a procedure requiring general anesthesia arrives at an ambulatory surgery center 30 minutes late for his preoperative assessment. The history and physical forwarded by his physician is brief. The nursing assessment is rushed and completed in a room full of distractions. As a result, neither the man nor his wife inform the nursing staff that certain anesthesia medications used during past operative procedures had changed his consciousness levels for a more prolonged period than normally expected.

His surgery, the final one scheduled for the day, begins and proceeds without mishap. In the postoperative recovery area, the man exceeds the "usual" stay by one hour. Staff members again are rushed and anxious to complete their work for the day. Because the man responds verbally and is able to dress with minimal assistance from his wife, staff members do not complete all steps in the postoperative assessment and discharge the man without identifying his residual mental confusion.

The man is wheeled out of the recovery area in a wheelchair and out the front door to where his wife is waiting. The wife leaves her husband sitting on a bench in front of the facility while she gets their car in an adjacent parking lot. After a minute or two, the man, not fully recovered from the effects of anesthesia, becomes confused and attempts to walk alone to the parking area. He steps into oncoming traffic, is struck by a vehicle, and sustains a fractured hip.

STRATEGY

Be Focused, Be Thorough

- Allow ample time to assess and reassess an individual's risk of falling.
- Consider all prescription and over-the-counter drugs and supplements the individual is taking.
- Use observation techniques and communicate with the individual or family for specific impairments.
- Frequently monitor the individual's status for changes in condition.
- Educate the care recipient and family members about fall prevention strategies to consider after the individual is discharged.

Incomplete Assessment

A 75-year-old surgical patient with dementia is placed on a surgical unit following a routine procedure on his foot that requires general anesthesia. The nursing staff provides him with a wheelchair and assumes that he is not at risk for injury because his room is close to and within clear view of the nursing station and only 10 feet from the elevator entrance. A member of the nursing staff is in the nursing station at all times.

At the end of the first morning on the unit, the man wheels himself to the far end of the unit where staff can no longer directly observe him. The man is found unconscious with multiple fractures after opening a closed fire door and falling down one flight of stairs in the wheelchair.

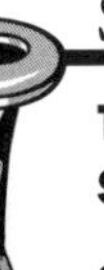

STRATEGY

Take Specific Measures for Specific Conditions

- Ensure continual observation of the care recipient.
- Completely assess and reassess an individual's risk of falling.
- Develop a care plan to address the specific condition of the care recipient.
- Follow processes related to dementia and appropriate care of individuals with dementia.
- Consider the physical environment and all the possibilities of a fall.

The first step in reducing falls is correctly and completely assessing and reassessing an individual's risk of falling. Many organizations build this risk assessment into the initial nursing assessment performed on admission. This assessment could include proper room or unit assignment for cognitively impaired individuals to areas where doors are locked or alarmed. As previously mentioned, risk factors include history of previous falls, mental status, communication, sensory and auditory deficits, medications, urinary alterations, and emotional upset.

The man in the second example above was at risk of falling due to cognitive impairment and residual effects of anesthesia. In a study conducted by Donna J. Conley, R.N., B.S.N., and colleagues in mid-1990, the risk factor of "impaired judgment" in fact contributed to the greatest relative risk of falling for hospitalized patients.[3]

A thorough reassessment process ensures that individualized interventions based on the initial assessment are meeting defined goals. Frequent monitoring allows team members to identify how the individual's status is changing. Observation of an individual's behavior is critical to reassessments conducted by nursing staff.

- *Thoroughly assess and reassess the individual for fall risk.* Health care leaders must ensure the assessment of each individual for fall risk as part of the interdisciplinary assessment process. Nurses assess for fall risk as part of the nursing assessment process. An initial assessment that fails to identify the individual's overall cognitive level, muscle strength, pain, toileting urgency and frequency, and ability to perform activities of daily living can lead to invalid conclusions about the individual's status. Assessing blood pressure while the individual is both sitting and standing for signs of insufficient blood flow and fainting is one effective proactive strategy. Thorough assessment enables nursing staff to suggest and implement a proactive approach to falls as part of the care planning and provision processes.
- *Consider all medications as part of the assessment and reassessment processes.* Nursing medication assessments and reassessments must take into account all prescription and over-the-counter drugs and supplements the individual is taking, any medication allergies, and history of substance abuse (including abuse of tranquilizers or other prescription drugs). Nurses can advocate for physician and pharmacologist review of the use of benzodiazepines, particularly those that are long acting, and limit the use of these psychotropic medications.

  Individuals with altered perception and cognition need aggressive and prompt assessment and regular reassessment from nursing staff. If an individual receiving behavioral health care services is not taking medications as prescribed, his or her alertness level may change and he or she may experience the psychiatric symptoms the medication alleviated when taken properly. Too much or too little insulin will change an individual's blood sugar level and can lead to disturbances in thought, as well as weakness, fainting, and dizziness. Some medications can cause dehydration in the elderly, which will also change mental status. These drugs are prescribed for various problems and can include blood pressure medication, cardiac drugs, and diuretics, to name a few. Sedation used during outpatient surgery and some diagnostic testing can place individuals at risk for falls if they are not allowed to rest and are not receiving close observation from nursing staff.

- *When indicated, use a combination of assessment techniques.* Use of different assessment techniques, such as observation or communication with the individual or family, help to provide as thorough an assessment as possible. For example, Conley mentions that she assesses individuals for impaired judgment through both observations and communication techniques. "I ask individuals to get out of the wheelchair and walk to the bed so that I can observe the level of support they need to walk," she says. Later in the assessment process, Conley asks individuals whether they need help in walking. If they say "no," but she observes otherwise, she determines that they exhibit impaired judgment and are considered "at risk" of falling. This impaired judgment could be the result of an individual's cognitive impairment (from the medication or another medical condition), or even from the individual's pride or sense of independence that prevents him or her from admitting that he or she needs help.
- *Assess according to established criteria and use a risk assessment tool.* Organization leaders must establish criteria specific to their care recipient population that place an individual at fall risk. Organizations frequently use an overall screening tool that includes fall risk, along with other assessments such as nutrition and skin integrity. Assessment tools help raise awareness of fall risk. Nurses need to use these tools whenever the care recipient becomes confused as the result of new medication or disruptions in daily routine. Nurses can help develop and implement tools specific to the population(s) served.
- *Obtain input from family members, and educate the care recipient and family about fall reduction strategies.* Communication with family members and significant others is critical to thorough assessment of fall risk. Staff should inform family members about factors that increase fall risk and inquire about the presence of any such factors. Educating the care recipient and family members about fall reduction strategies can help to reduce risk in the health care organization and after the individual is discharged. Techniques to improve strength and balance are particularly critical. In some organizations, physical therapists will provide such education, which the nursing staff can reinforce.
- *Reassess regularly to ensure success of interventions and decreased risk of falls.* Among other changes, medication changes—including drug additions and increased or decreased dosages—create the need for vigilant monitoring for possible new side effects. A new medication added to an individual's current medication regimen can cause dizziness, sedation, or some other symptom that places the individual at an increased risk for falls. Regular nursing staff scheduled reassessment, in addition to assessment and monitoring for behaviors indicating impaired judgment—particularly if the individual has had any sort of procedure involving anesthesia—can

reduce the risk of falls. Staff monitoring of laboratory values for potential toxicity levels, which can cause changes in mental and physical ability, can also help reduce falls.

- *Increase awareness of processes related to dementia and appropriate care of individuals with dementia.* In unfamiliar surroundings, individuals with dementia may experience an increased level of confusion at dusk and night that is called "sundowning." This is a high-risk time of day for falls for individuals with dementia. Staff can develop care plans to address the assessed need to increase fall reduction measures at this time of day. Activities to redirect and divert the individual's attention can be provided, such as music, visitors, or pet therapy, as appropriate. Additional information regarding care for individuals with Alzheimer's, one form of dementia, can be found through the Alzheimer's Association at http://www.alz.org.

Root Cause Example: Unsafe Environment of Care

An organization provides subacute care to individuals with AIDS, many of whom have AIDS–related dementia. Care is provided in a unit on the third floor of a multistory building. Care recipients generally are ambulatory, except those in the final disease stage. Unit windows open 10 inches.

During early morning rounds, the nursing staff are not able to locate one individual. A nurse notes that one of the windows in the individual's room is open as far as it can be. Simultaneously, a visitor finds the man outside the facility, having fallen three floors while attempting to leave the building. He was so thin that he was able to work his way out the window, and so confused that he did not realize that his own room was on the third floor. Staff who installed the windows were not aware of how thin and emaciated AIDS patients could become. Although the fall does not prove fatal, the individual has significant injuries requiring an extended acute care stay.

STRATEGY

Specialize and Prioritize

- Have specifically trained staff make regular environmental rounds to check for possible hazards.
- Improve environmental assessment by staff on the AIDS unit.
- Increase education of the environmental and safety staff of the conditions of individuals with AIDS.

Organization leaders must ensure planning for a safe environment and implementation of a safety plan. Safety efforts should include making regular environmental rounds to check for possible hazards such as those that could contribute to falls. Individuals conducting these rounds should be trained to ensure safety compliance in all areas, including care units.

The participation of nurses and other staff members on environmental rounds can also help to reduce potential environmental hazards. Nurses are well equipped to identify problems that could lead high-risk care recipients to fall while trying to ambulate without assistance. Improved environmental assessment by nursing staff on the AIDS unit described above could have helped to reduce the risk of the man's fall while attempting to elope. Increased education of the environmental and safety staff about the conditions of individuals with AIDS might also have helped to reduce the risk of this fall.

SIDEBAR 2-1

Environmental Checklist to Identify Fall Risks

1. Temperature of the room is comfortable.
2. The room is free of odors.
3. Ventilation is adequate.
4. Noise level is acceptable.
5. Lighting is adequate and minimizes glare.
6. Floors are free of clutter, and are clean and dry.
7. The room is clean.
8. The room is free of hazards (for example, bed cranks are in, no spills, electrical cords out of the way).
9. A bedside table is available.
10. Handrails are present and secure in the toilet area.
11. Call light system is in working order and accessible to the care recipient (check response time).
12. Bed wheels are locked or in blocks.
13. Closet and shelf space are accessible to the care recipient.
14. Equipment (for example, lifts, wheelchairs, walkers) is in good repair.[4]

- *Help ensure basic environmental safety.* Although housekeeping staff are ultimately responsible for keeping the care environment clean and tidy, nurses can play a key role in ensuring a safe environment of care. Areas used by care recipients must be clean and free of clutter. They also must be free of spills and loose cords or wires that could trip the care recipient, staff, or visitors. Slippery floors can lead to falls in all types of health care settings. A nurse who is aware of floor conditions, such as wetness caused by people bringing moisture from outside, or a housekeeping person not mopping floors in the correct manner so there is a dry path to walk on, can take actions to address the unsafe conditions. They also can advise care recipients and family members to take extra caution. Environmental checklists, such as the one shown in Sidebar 2-1, serve as a guide to identifying fall risks.

  Equipment used by care recipients, such as wheelchairs, walkers, and canes, must be in proper repair. Proper-fitting footwear allows for safe ambulating. Another checklist, developed by nursing staff, is often used when conducting weekly environmental rounds to identify and prioritize problems that could lead to falls (see Sidebar 2-2, page 40).
- *Be knowledgeable about the organization's preventive maintenance program, and be vigilant about equipment needs and concerns.* Nursing staff should know how to check equipment used by individuals receiving care for safety considerations and know how to notify maintenance of equipment needs and concerns. Organization leaders must ensure staff training about how to identify unsafe equipment, as well as the required steps to remove unsafe equipment from use.
- *Be particularly alert to unsafe bathrooms.* As mentioned earlier, falls frequently occur in bathrooms or on the way to the bathrooms in all types of health care settings. Older individuals who have not been able to go to

SIDEBAR 2-2

Selections on Environmental Strategies

Lighting

- Provide proper illumination in the environment and adjust to the individual needs of patient and residents.
- Provide light switches that allow a person to increase or decrease illumination levels as desired.
- Extra (strategic) lighting may be needed in certain locations such as the bedroom, path from the bed to the bathroom, and toilet area.
- Consider using motion-sensor bathroom lighting.
- Use good floor-level night-lights (avoid night-lights that merely create shadows and glare).
- Quality of lighting is important for safe ambulation (for example, full spectrum fluorescent light is more effective than incandescent lighting for overall illumination of the environment).

Floor Surfaces

- Minimize highly polished floors. In addition to being a slip hazard, buffing and polishing can cause reflected glare giving the floor an appearance of being wet or slick. This may lead to the care recipient being in fear of ambulation and gait changes.
- Consider using slip-resistant flooring and slip-resistant adhesive strips in areas such as the floor next to the sink and toilet.
- In certain settings (for example, long term care facilities), low-pile carpeting may be considered.

Hallways

- Avoid clutter (for example, medicine, laundry, food carts, cleaning equipment, wheelchairs) in hallways.
- As patients or residents may become fatigued in ambulating long hallways on the way to reach the nurses station, dining rooms, and so forth, consider providing "rest stops," or chairs strategically placed every 20 to 30 feet.

Handrail Support

- Provide handrails for support and ensure proper height from floor (26 to 36 inches) and design (for example, round grip).

Bed Height, Support, and Mattresses

- Keep beds in their lowest position when feasible.
- Use height adjustable "hi-low" beds or fixed low-deck-height beds where applicable.
- Consider providing a bed footboard to assist patients and residents in transferring in and out of bed or in ambulating about the bedroom.
- Mattresses should be firm enough to support necessary safe bed transfers.

Bed Side Rails and Wheels

- Routine use of bed side rails (when applicable) is still a standard practice in many hospitals.
- Evaluate their safe application carefully.
- As care recipients may attempt to climb over bed rails, consider the use of half bed side rails (compared to full-length rails) as the standard.
- Use good bed wheel-locking systems such as a combination swivel-and-wheel brake.
- Nonslip adhesive strips placed underneath the bed wheels may reduce further slippage.

Bed Alarm Systems

- The significant decline in the use of mechanical and chemical restraints to reduce high-risk care recipient falls has stimulated the proliferation of bed alarm systems. These are designed to warn nursing staff that care recipients who should not attempt to leave their bed unassisted are doing so.
- Evaluate and choose alarm systems based on such features as loudness, built-in time delays or ease of use.[5]

the bathroom due to long waits for tests, crowded bathrooms, or delayed toileting assistance may not be able to control bladder functions. The result may be dribbled urine while getting on or off the toilet. This represents a safety hazard. Nonskid floor coverings in toilet areas can help reduce fall risk and can be recommended by nursing staff. Nursing staff can be aware when individuals may need additional assistance with getting on and off the toilet. Some individuals are too embarrassed to request help, particularly if they are in an outpatient area such as the laboratory or X-ray room, and can be asked whether they need assistance in a manner that ensures their privacy.

- *Use safety devices properly.* When properly used, bed alarms, self-latching devices on utility rooms, exit alarms, "low beds" for those at risk for falls, locking bed wheels, and handrails can significantly reduce the risk of falls in every organization. Some organizations use bracelets worn by individuals at risk of falling as an extra precaution to reduce the risk of individuals leaving the appropriate area. The bracelet triggers a door alarm, alerting staff if the individual approaches and attempts to open the door.
- *Use fall reduction environment of care protocols established by the organization.* Staff should identify individuals at high risk of falling and provide additional environmental safety measures as outlined by organizational leaders. Protocols might address such items as not allowing postsurgical patients to be up and about without supervision or staff assistance for a defined number of hours following surgery, and encouraging family members to visit in "shifts" to help monitor the individual's status. When designing space, some organizations adopt a pod configuration in which the nursing station is located in the center of radiating rooms. Individuals at high risk of falling and others requiring maximum observation receive beds closer to the nursing station.

Root Cause Examples: Inadequate Care Planning and Provision

Incomplete Care Planning

A man is admitted for behavioral health treatment. His physician's history and physical do not identify a previous allergy to a particular medication. The man's guardian briefly states that, in the past, the man had been on numerous medications for his psychiatric condition and that he may have had reactions to some of the drugs. Because the information was vague at best, the nurse does not identify or document any allergies and completes the man's plan of care without addressing past medication sensitivity. The psychiatric resident on call orders lithium after reviewing the man's record. Within four hours, the man is found unconscious in the day area of the facility, having fallen and broken an arm and hip.

STRATEGY

Individual Care, Team Approach

- Conduct a thorough medication assessment of the care recipient on admission.
- Document medication allergies and drug reactions that may increase fall risk.
- Ensure a multifactorial, interdisciplinary approach to assessment and reassessment.
- Communicate the care recipient's condition across disciplines.

Inadequate Care Provision

A home health nurse visits a 69-year-old woman recovering from hip replacement surgery. The nurse's role is to monitor the condition of the woman's hip incision, reinforce exercises ordered by the physical therapist, and help the woman learn to use a new walker recommended by the physical therapist for ambulation. During her first visit, the nurse assesses the woman and her needs. The nurse does not follow the care plan and assists the woman with ambulation, providing contact guard assistance rather than helping with the walker. The woman had used the walker prior to surgery, but during her hospitalization a neighbor had borrowed it. Unfortunately, the neighbor changed the walker's height and, having damaged one of the four wheels, replaced it with a smaller wheel. After the nurse leaves, the woman attempts to use the walker and falls, breaking her arm during the fall. Review of the nurse's narrative notes confirms the nurse's failure to redirect the woman to ambulate using the walker and to ensure that the walker was in working order and appropriately fitted.

STRATEGY

Consider All Conditions

- Assess the condition of all walking aids and equipment.
- Ensure that reduction strategies are highly individualized.
- Communicate and document a care recipient's condition across the continuum of care.

The first example demonstrates the importance of a thorough medication assessment on admission of individuals receiving care. Undocumented medication allergies place an individual at increased risk of adverse drug reactions and increased risk of falls.

As demonstrated in other examples, the reduction of falls requires a multifactorial, interdisciplinary approach. After an individual has been identified as at risk for falls, a multidisciplinary team should begin the care planning process and provide care according to the care plan. The nursing care plan is generally the first step in this process and is followed by additional disciplines, as determined by the care recipient's needs. Medical, nursing, pharmacy, and physical/occupational therapy staff participate in many care settings.

For example, interventions for an individual at risk of falling due to poor vision include balance and gait training by physical therapists, low-vision aids from optometrists, and environmental safety assessment by nursing and occupational therapy staff. Interventions for a person at risk of falling due to foot problems may include foot care by podiatrists or orthopedic staff, as well as adaptive devices and proper shoes from occupational therapy and nursing staff. Interventions for an individual at risk of falling due to taking multiple medications include selection of medications that are least associated with fall risk, prescription of the lowest effective dose with the shortest action by pharmacy, and medical staff monitoring by nursing staff.

The role of pharmacists and prescribers in team-oriented care planning is particularly critical due to the high correlation between falls and medication use. Pharmacists can identify specific drugs and drug categories that are associated with such fall risk factors as confusion, orthostatic hypotension, and dizziness. Pharmacists must alert interdisciplinary team members of the potential adverse risks associated with particular medications and work closely with physicians to determine whether continuation of the medication(s) in question is desirable given associated risks and treatment goals.

They not only play a key role in educating nurses and physical and occupational therapists about symptoms to look for in individuals taking medications that increase the risk of falls, but also alert team members about specific monitoring parameters.

In health care settings, too often the process of reviewing care recipients for their risk of fall does not include a pharmacist. According to some medical professionals, however, a review of a care recipient's medication by a pharmacist can dramatically reduce the likelihood that a care recipient will fall and be injured.[6]

In assessing medications, a pharmacist is able to look for those that increase the risk of falls, or combinations that may increase the risk of falls. Along with his colleagues, Mark J. Haumschild, M.S., Pharm.D, cardiovascular/thrombosis scientific manager with Aventis Pharmaceuticals in Seminole, Florida, and consultant pharmacist for Morton Plant Mease Health Care (MPMHC) in Clearwater, Florida, implemented a systematic review process at MPMHC, a rehabilitation center, that resulted in 47% fewer falls in a one-year period (October 1, 2000, to September 30, 2001). The group estimated that this reduction in falls saved the center $308,000 in health care costs.[7]

"We decided to develop a program where we looked at each resident's drug use more intensely," Haumschild explains. "We wanted to make recommendations for discontinuing a drug, changing the dosage, or switching to a different drug for that particular care recipient, based on comorbidities."

This simple, effective process begins when a new resident is admitted. Upon admission, the staff at the rehabilitation center faxes a list of medications and dosages for Haumschild to review. In most cases, the care recipient's medications were reviewed within 24 hours of admission. This process supports the National Patient Safety Goal for reconciling medications.

In an effort to study the effectiveness of the process, called the fall-focused pharmaceutical intervention program (FFPIP), Haumschild randomly selected 200 care recipients from the preintervention and postintervention periods. A data analysis found that the number of care recipient falls was reduced in the postintervention group by 47%, resulting in an estimated future savings of $7.74 per care recipient per day. The data also showed that the use of several classes of medication decreased in the postintervention period as follows:

- Cardiovascular agents were reduced by 10.7%.
- Analgesics were reduced by 6.3%.
- Psychoactive drugs were reduced by 18.2%.
- Sedatives and hypnotics were reduced by 13.9%.[7]

From this research emerged a profile of the type of care recipient most at risk for falls. According to the profile, care recipients most likely to fall were males greater than 76 years of age who had a cardiovascular or orthopedic-related diagnosis. These care recipients were also taking analgesics, cardiovascular agents, and central nervous system agents.

"The process was based on us going over each care recipient's record and either reducing drug dosages or modifying their therapy in some way," Haumschild says. "That won't work unless you have the support of their physicians, but we found that physicians were very supportive."

Haumschild also worked with nurses at the rehabilitation center in implementing new recommendations for watching care recipients more closely. Because a sudden drop in blood pressure can lead to falls, these recommendations were based partly on education about how a care recipient's blood pressure can be affected by a change in body position. Education efforts included not only nurses, but most of the center's staff, including housekeeping, transportation, and therapists.

"Simply educating them about blood pressure changes and position made them much more alert to risky situations," Haumschild says. "That was part of what led to the overall reduction in falls."

According to Haumschild, the success of the intervention program could be replicated in any health care setting. As a consultant pharmacist not involved in actively dispensing drugs, Haumschild noted that dispensing pharmacists might find it more difficult to incorporate medication reviews into their work loads. In this case, he suggested a system in which the dispensing pharmacist reviews the care recipient's prescription medications when drug prescriptions are filled. This, he says, may lessen the burden of having a list of medications sent for review while trying to fill orders.

"The moment the drug is dispensed is a tremendous opportunity to make a difference because they can see that the care recipient is on certain drugs and make recommendations," Haumschild says. "They can affect the fall risk almost immediately."

The rehabilitation center recently added pharmaceutical review as part of its monthly risk management committee meeting. Made up of a risk manager and representatives from several departments, the committee now includes Haumschild as well. With falls as a priority, the committee reviews a couple of injury cases each month. Assessing the care recipient's medication regimen is a vital aspect of their effort to determine whether the injury could have been avoided.

"The pharmacist is usually not involved enough in that effort, actually looking at care recipients in the fall evaluations," Haumschild says. "You usually have nurses and physicians involved in assessing fall risk at admission, but that's also where the pharmacist should get involved."

Tailor fall reduction strategies to the individual's unique needs. Reduction strategies must be highly individualized. A care recipient's family members may be able to provide information on the individual habits and activities that could help to individualize these strategies. Some combined assessment and care planning tools enable nursing staff to select appropriate interventions, based on the individual's risk level. In some cases, staff may need to adjust medications; in other cases, walkers, assistance, or anything in between may be needed. For example, frequent toileting is an effective intervention for cognitively impaired individuals and those on diuretics. "The former don't realize that they need help in getting to the toilet," notes Jane E. Mahoney, M.D., assistant professor of medicine in the geriatric section of the University of Wisconsin Medical School. Falls on the way to the bathroom account for a large proportion of all falls in hospitals. Assisting with toileting when individuals receive diuretic medications, tranquilizers, or sedatives reduces fall risk. Also, giving diuretics to individuals while they are awake and active rather than before they go to sleep can help to reduce falls that can occur when tired individuals must get out of bed to use the bathroom.

In numerous instances, falls result when an individual tries to get out of bed. In some long term care facilities, staff place mattresses on the floor so residents have less distance to fall if they roll off the bed. Organizations are also beginning to purchase electric beds that allow the bed height to decrease six to eight inches from the floor. For individuals with Huntington's disease, which causes random, spasmodic movements while individuals are sleeping and awake, adult-size enclosed beds are used with success. One side rail can be left in a low position and a large mat placed by the bed.

Help to ensure the provision of timely care. Timeliness of care has a significant impact on reducing fall risk. Many care recipients fall on the way to requesting nurse or other caregiver assistance. They may attempt to walk without required help when they are trying to alert the nursing staff to their need for toileting or pain control medication. By tracking the amount of time taken to answer call lights and decreasing response time, a number of organizations have noted a decreased number of falls linked to decreased response time.[8] Improved and standardized call systems can reduce fall likelihood, as can administering pain medications before transfers or ambulation to decrease discomfort and allow for increased mobility and toileting according to a schedule established with the care recipient.

Recognize fall risk associated with restraint use and eliminate restraint use whenever possible.[9] Studies conducted in the long term care community in the 1990s[10] indicated that, although the number of falls might have been higher initially in a restraint-free environment, injury severity declined significantly.[11] Restraint can increase the risk of harm and actually cause harm to individuals. Because muscles are not being used, prolonged use of restraints can decrease an individual's muscle strength and thereby increase the likelihood of falls when the individual is not in restraints. In addition, the use of restraints can increase fall risk as individuals try to escape their restraint. For example, an individual trying to get out of bed with full bed rails might experience a more serious fall than if split bed rails were used. Between 1985 and 1999, 315 incidents of individuals getting caught, trapped, entangled, or strangled in beds with rails, resulting in death or injury, were reported to the Food and Drug Administration.[12]

The Hospital Bed Safety Workgroup, with representatives from more than 25 health care organizations, including the Joint Commission and companies providing products and services to health care organizations, encourages health care organizations to assess care recipients' needs and to provide safe care without restraints. A half rail in the up position at the head of the bed may help reduce the risk of individuals rolling out of the bed, and a lowered half rail at the foot of the bed will let them get out of bed when needed. If individuals should not get out of bed without assistance, bed alarms can be used to alert staff to the individuals' movement. Alternatives to bed rails suggested by the group appear in Sidebar 2-3, page 46.

Effective alternatives to restraints exist in all health care settings. Nursing staff should be knowledgeable about alternate safe and appropriate interventions. If restraints are necessary, nursing staff should ensure that they are properly used. The example on page 46 offers evidence that alternatives to restraints can reduce care recipient falls.

Understanding the root causes of care recipient falls and considering various intervention strategies designed to reduce them will better prepare health care organizations and staff to develop an effective fall risk assessment plan. Keeping this in mind, the following chapter outlines the aspects and approaches to risk assessment and stresses the importance of proper risk assessment in any comprehensive fall reduction program.

SIDEBAR 2-3

Alternatives to Using Bed Rails

In most cases, care recipients can remain safely in bed without the use of bed rails. The following ideas can be implemented to avoid using bed rails:

- Check on care recipients frequently. Often, close observation can reduce falls better than bed rails.
- Use adjustable beds that can be raised and lowered to make it easier for care recipients to get in and out of beds and easier for staff to assist in this process.
- Use transfer or mobility aids.
- For individuals at high risk of falls, put mats next to the bed to absorb impact when falls do occur. However, make sure that the mats do not increase the risk of falls due to tripping or uneven footing.
- Identify reasons why individuals get out of bed, including hunger, thirst, bathroom needs, restlessness, insomnia, and pain. Try to meet these needs on a predictable schedule that care recipients are aware of and have input into.[13]

EXAMPLE 2-1

U.S. Department of Veterans Affairs (VA) Facility Reduces Restraint Use, Boosts Alternatives

Many health care organizations rely on the use of restraints to reduce the risk of their patients pulling out tubes, being combative, or doing anything that might interfere with their care. Yet the use of restraints can also lead to an increase in falls. As a result, organizations have begun to look at alternatives to restraint use that reduce fall risk and improve safety, and have successfully implemented efforts toward finding alternatives to restraint use that ultimately led to fewer falls.

Identifying the Problem

An elderly patient with severe dementia was a client in restraints at the William S. Middleton Memorial VA Medical Center's acute psychiatric unit. He was so cognitively impaired that he could not communicate his most basic needs. The nurses did not know how best to care for the patient other than to keep him restrained to reduce his risk of falling and injuring himself.

After a case conference, the nurses placed the patient on a toileting program and a pain management program, as well as on increased observation. A bed alarm and a chair alarm were used to alert nurses to his attempts to ambulate without assistance. Within days, he grew stronger, became less agitated, responded to verbal cues, and was taken out of restraints entirely. Within a week, the man was placed in an Alzheimer's unit in a nursing home where he could receive more appropriate care. Previously, nursing homes had refused to take him because he was in restraints and his behavior was uncontrolled.

"That was a turning point," says Bill Keuler, R.N., program manager for hospital-based mental

(continued)

EXAMPLE 2-1 (continued)

health at the VA Medical Center in Madison, Wisconsin. "The nurses began to see that they could be effective in managing patients like this using alternatives and trying different care strategies."

That incident occurred a few months after the nurse managers' group, under the direction of the nurse executive, began concerted efforts to reduce restraint use in the medical center. It was around the same time that the Madison facility began participating in a VA fall reduction program aimed at reducing falls and injuries due to falls. As part of this eight-month quality improvement collaborative, teams tracked fall and injury rates monthly as they implemented a variety of interventions.

Meanwhile, the organization continued to monitor restraint use as it had done for years, without affecting much change in practice, says Keuler. The culture within the institution was that "falls happen and nothing can be done about them," which is a commonly held belief throughout health care organizations, he notes. Until recently, that attitude was traditionally reinforced in many nursing schools, where nurses were trained on how to place restraints and not on how to use alternatives, adds Keuler.

Delving Deeper

In late 1999, a performance improvement project examining restraint use found that many patients requiring restraints were suffering from delirium associated with alcohol withdrawal. Nurses were using restraints to protect patients from falling or wandering. In many cases, patients were going undiagnosed and consequently not being effectively treated for withdrawal. They became more delirious over time, resulting in increased restraint use. Patients who tried pulling out IVs and various tubes were also restrained, as were patients who wandered as a result of confusion.

After learning this, Keuler organized four half-day workshops on the management of alcohol withdrawal. Additionally, a tool for identifying patients experiencing alcohol withdrawal was modified and adopted, enabling staff to better recognize the underlying cause of the delirium. As a result, restraint rates started to decline.

As part of the fall reduction team's efforts to focus on the environment, an aggregated review of the fall incident reports from the previous year showed that there was a pattern of patient falls. They were falling in a small area around the exit side of the bed, says Bruce Kramer, R.N., B.S.N., nurse manager, who headed up the fall reduction program at Madison. Through patient and staff interviews, he learned that patients often fell because they were standing up either to move toward the bathroom or use the urinal. The other scenario was that they slipped after spilling something on the floor and had nothing to hold onto.

Finding Restraint Alternatives

Kramer arranged for an equipment manufacturer to present a half-day workshop focusing on restraint alternatives and the hazards of restraining patients. In 2000 he ordered several thousand dollars' worth of restraint alternatives, including the following:

(continued)

EXAMPLE 2-1 (continued)

- Bed exit alarms
- Chair exit alarms
- Voice alarms telling the patient not to get up because a nurse would come by shortly to help
- Freedom splints (sleeves that fit over the forearm and upper arm) to reduce the risk of the patient pulling out tubes
- Torso supports to maintain the patient's posture and positioning
- Mitts to keep the patient from pulling out IVs and nasogastric tubes
- Antiskid floor mats that absorb fluids and food
- Antislip footwear

Many of the equipment pieces were used in "safe room" setups that were piloted on a 22-bed general medical telemetry unit. When patients scored high on a fall scale that was implemented to identify patients at risk for falls, they were assigned to a safe room.

Throughout 2000, restraint alternatives were pilot tested on one of the three medical/surgical units. Those that proved successful were introduced throughout the organization. Staff nurses were trained on how to use the equipment. Additionally, providing care in a restraint-free environment is addressed in educational sessions, staff orientation, and staff competency, the latter of which is part of the annual review.

It was shortly after the fall reduction team began investigating restraint alternatives that the two efforts—reducing restraint use and reducing injuries to falls—came together. "When Bruce's team started focusing on how to reduce falls, we found some of the equipment he was using in the falls reduction program were things we could use to replace restraints," says Keuler. "Before, all we could do is tell our staff nurses that they shouldn't be using restraints. This was the first time we had some alternatives to offer to them."

Collecting the Data

Documenting restraint use was made simpler with the use of electronic orders that automatically print out a flow sheet when a physician puts in a written order for restraints. Nurses no longer have to fill out any reports or logs; they simply fill out the restraint flow sheet, which makes tracking restraint use much easier, and document what restraint alternatives were attempted, notes Kramer.

A data management clerk enters data from the flow sheets onto a spreadsheet. All nurse managers and nurse executives have access to the data, which is compared month to month, and is broken down by shift and by days of the week. In addition, a physician order for restraints automatically generates an alert to all the nurse managers that there is a new patient on restraints. They review those patients on a 24-hour basis and also review the flow sheets. Although nurse managers can access the data at any time, they conduct a formal review monthly. A quarterly report is sent to the Coordination of Care Committee, comprised of allied service chiefs.

The data are so precise that Kramer noted a trend on his floor in which a few nurses on the

(continued)

EXAMPLE 2-1 (continued)

night shift continued to restrain patients who were experiencing alcohol withdrawal and were at high risk for falls. He was able to identify which nurses were doing so and with positive encouragement was able to reeducate them. "Some nurses just didn't believe that they could protect patients from injury if they didn't tie them down," says Kramer.

Restraint Rates Fall

In fact, they can fall. Restraint use fell from 2.27% on the medical/surgical units in fiscal 1999 to 0.35% in the first quarter of 2003. It dropped from 8.56% on the psychiatric unit in 1999 to 0.24% in the first quarter of 2003. Restraint use also declined from 24.65% in the intensive care unit (ICU) in 1999 to 20.25% in the first quarter of 2003. When the fall reduction project concluded, falls and minor injuries had been reduced by 18% on the pilot unit, with no major injuries reported. Since then, the overall fall rate has remained steady, but major injuries dropped 50% and minor injuries declined 10% throughout the medical center.

Lessons Learned

The Madison VA offers the following tips for finding alternatives to restraint use and reducing falls:

- Educate staff on how to create a "culture of safety."
- Provide equipment that can serve as an alternative(s) to restraints.
- Have champions on each unit to take the lead.
- Take a nonpunitive approach.
- Keep administrative oversight at the unit level by the nurse manager.
- Make data collection easy, to facilitate reporting and analysis.

The current focus is on cutting restraint use in the ICU, says Kramer. Beginning in 2003, nurses required a physician's order to use restraint protocols in the ICU. Another area of focus is repeat fallers, that is, patients who have had two or more reported falls. In addition, beds with built-in alarms are being evaluated. Based on the literature, they may have a significant impact on the use of restraints and reduction of falls, Kramer says.

The biggest hurdle to reducing restraint use was getting buy-in from his colleagues, says Kramer. "The quickest way to clear a room was to bring up restraint usage. It was a thankless, difficult endeavor for many years," he notes. "But our current success has been fulfilling for the staff nurses because they feel they are providing better patient care."[14]

References

1. Health and Safety Commission: *Organizing for Safety: Third Report of the Human Factors Study Group of ACSNI.* Sudbury, UK: HSE Books, 1993.
2. Joint Commission Resources: Catch them before they fall with multidisciplinary care plans. *Jt Comm Benchmark* 2:1–3, Dec. 2000.
3. Conley D., Schults A.A., Selvin R.: The challenge of predicting patients at risk for falling: Development of the Conley Scale. *MEDSURG Nursing* 8:348–354, Dec. 1999.
4. Joint Commission Resources: *Using Hospital Standards to Prevent Sentinel Events.* Oakbrook Terrace, IL: Joint Commission on Accreditation of Healthcare Organizations, 2001, p. 120.
5. Tideiksaar R.: *Falls in Older People: Prevention and Management,* 3rd ed. Baltimore: Health Professions Press, 2002.
6. Healthcare Risk Management: Pharmacists meds review may reduce patient falls. *Healthcare Risk Management* p. 81, Jul. 2003.
7. Haumschild M.J., et al.: Clinical and economic outcomes of a fall-focused pharmaceutical intervention program. *Am J Health-Syst Pharm* 60:1029–1032, May 2003.
8. Joint Commission Resources: *Using Hospital Standards to Prevent Sentinel Events.* Oakbrook Terrace, IL: Joint Commission on Accreditation of Healthcare Organizations, 2001, p. 114.
9. Strumpf N.E., Evans L.K.: Alternatives to physical restraints. *J Ger Nurs* 18:4, 1992.
10. Evans L.K., Strumpf N.E., Williams C.: Redefining a standard of care for frail older people: Alternatives to routine physical restraint. In Katz P., Kane R., Mezey R. (eds.): *Advances in Long Term Care.* New York: Springer, 1991, pp. 81–108.
11. Evans L.K., Strumpf N.E.: Myths about elder restraint. *J of Nurs Scholarship* 22: 124–128, Summer 1990.
12. Hospital Bed Safety Workgroup: *A Guide to Bed Safety: Bed Rails in Hospitals, Nursing Homes, and Home Health Care: The Facts.* U.S. Food and Drug Administration. Oct. 11, 2000. http://www.fda.gov/cdrh/beds (accessed Mar. 12, 2005).
13. Adapted from Hospital Bed Safety Workgroup: *A Guide to Bed Safety: Bed Rails in Hospitals, Nursing Homes, and Home Health Care:* The Facts. U.S. Food and Drug Administration. Oct. 11, 2000. http://www.fda.gov/cdrh/beds (accessed Mar. 12, 2005).
14. Joint Commission Resources: VA Facility Reduces Restraint Use, Boosts Alternatives. *Joint Commission Perspectives on Patient Safety* 3:7–8, Jul. 2003.

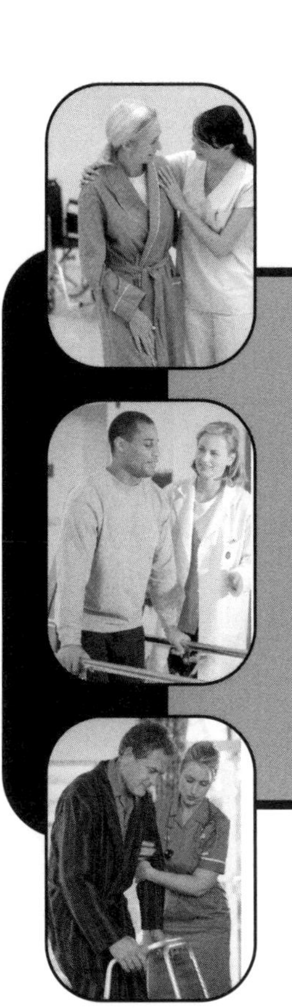

CHAPTER 3

The Elements of Effective Fall Risk Assessment

A 42-year-old man with alcoholic cirrhosis, blood clotting, low platelets, and a history of hemorrhaging from falls was admitted. The neurosurgery service drained the clotting blood via burr holes. During the first week of hospitalization, the patient received a total of 45 units of fresh frozen plasma in an effort to minimize the chances of expansion of the clots. The patient showed continued improvement and was transferred from the intensive care unit to the step-down unit.

The patient was identified as being a fall risk. The following precautions were taken:

- *The bed was placed in the lowest possible position.*
- *The bedside call button was made immediately accessible.*
- *The patient was explicitly told to call the nurse if anything was needed.*
- *The patient was placed in an area close to nursing staff.*
- *The bed alarm was activated.*

The patient stated that he did not want to be physically restrained, and staff believed him to be competent. The next evening, the patient attempted to get out of the bed and fell to the floor.

In this case, was staff fully educated on the care recipient's risk factors? Did staff follow the steps of thorough assessment? Did staff take an interdisciplinary approach in risk assessment? Did staff choose appropriate risk assessment tools in this case? Did staff initiate a care plan based on a complete assessment?

For many health care professionals, assessment tools are seen as the anchor of any effective fall reduction program. The results of many expert studies identifying risk factors of care recipients in acute care settings indicate that few patients or residents were excluded from being identified as "at risk." Although care recipient falls have been reported as the largest single category of reported incidents in hospitals,[1,2] fall reduction programs in many health care organizations do not take full advantage of the risk assessment process. "Some programs and instruments aimed at identifying the patient at risk of falling have been used even though they were not developed from the patient assessment, were not tested with control groups, and were not assessed for reliability and validity," according to Janice M. Morse, Ph.D., F.A.A.N.[3]

In responding to the fall example above and the questions it provokes, this chapter makes a case for the importance of the risk assessment process in persistently combating the problem of care recipient falls. It also serves as a guide to the characteristics and approaches that help make fall risk assessment such a valuable tool to health care organizations and the individuals they serve. Among the areas and issues covered are the importance of an interdisciplinary team, the proper education and communication of staff, the variety of risk assessment tools, and the necessary considerations in choosing the appropriate assessment tool.

Through her studies, Morse has identified that care recipient falls within an institution are not simply random events. They are patterned and predictable occurrences that are preventable.[3] Factors that place residents at risk for falls include a previous history of falls, cognitive impairment, impaired balance or mobility, musculoskeletal problems, chronic diseases, nutritional problems, and use of multiple medications. Residents of long term care facilities are often elderly and frail, and are thus at increased risk of falling. Because many of these residents are cognitively impaired, they often do not realize their level of impairment and are therefore not able to take the extra care needed to protect themselves from falling.

Thorough risk assessment enables staff to suggest and implement a proactive approach to reducing falls as part of the care planning and provision process. "Initial and ongoing comprehensive interdisciplinary assessments enable staff to look for the red flags that could prevent a fall risk," explains Victoria Christian, surveyor for the Joint Commission's long term care and hospital accreditation programs. An initial assessment that fails to identify the individual's overall cognitive level, muscle strength, pain, and ability to perform activities of daily living can lead to invalid conclusions about the individual's status.

There are many important ingredients to an effective fall risk assessment process—including an unwavering commitment to the ongoing education of staff and consistent communication among staff. Many health care experts agree that the strength of these elements depends on the contribution of an organization's interdisciplinary team.

A Team Approach to Risk Assessment

No matter the setting, health care leaders must ensure that assessing and reassessing each individual for fall risk is part of the interdisciplinary assessment process. "Ideally, an organization should appoint an interdisciplinary team to design or select tools to use with specific populations," according to Joint Commission surveyor Anne Piper, R.N., M.S. "They should do a literature search and review standards of care and benchmarks for those populations. They should also look at historical data and involve both clinical and support staff in areas within the organization where falls have been a problem."

After internal examination of the organization and an external review of existing literature, the interdisciplinary fall team can begin the work of establishing best-practice standards for a comprehensive fall risk assessment tool that will assist its health care team in gathering care recipient information related to falls on admission to the hospital and on an ongoing basis.[4]

A health care organization's interdisciplinary team is responsible for planning care and services for each care recipient, based on identified needs. The interdisciplinary team can evaluate how clinical and environmental factors intersect to place the care recipient at risk and then identify interventions to minimize that risk. The team monitors the ongoing cognitive abilities and determines the effect of medications on the care recipient's ability to follow directions and maneuver the environment safely.

Team Members

The members of the team may vary, depending on the care needs. In addition to the care recipient or designated family members, the team includes the attending physician, who is responsible for coordinating the medical plan of care, and other clinical staff such as nursing staff, therapy staff, and the dietitian.

According to the National Center for Patient Safety Falls Toolkit, an interdisciplinary fall team should include staff with administrative and direct care functions.

The following clinical staff should be included:

1. Falls clinical nurse specialist (or similar position)
2. Nurse managers (one from each area: outpatient care, acute care, and extended care)
3. Nursing assistants/licensed practical nurses (LPNs) (one from acute care and one from extended care; could involve two from each area of care with each person rotating to attend meetings)
4. Pharmacist (one or two, depending on work load and staffing levels)
5. Occupational therapist or physical therapist
6. Physician/nurse practitioner (may be full participant on the team or act as a resource for the team)

Nonclinical staff should include the following:

1. Patient safety manager/quality management coordinator (or similar position)
2. Facility management manager
3. Supply procurement and distribution manager
4. Biotechnology manager (optional)
5. Transportation manager (optional; one facility added this person due to the number of falls occurring while care recipients were being transported)

The responsibilities of each team member should be clearly defined in policy or in the team procedures or charter.

Clinical staff responsibilities should include the following:

- *Falls clinical nurse specialist.* Not all facilities have a falls clinical nurse specialist. Some facilities have a particular nurse manager, generally in the long term or extended care wards, who has an interest in falls and fall-related injury reduction. This person will generally facilitate team meetings, ensure that fall reduction measures are being used (this is also the responsibility of the entire team), and elicit comments from staff regarding the program and other fall-related activities.

- *Nurse managers from outpatient, acute, and extended care.* Nurse managers are an important part of the fall interdisciplinary team. Due to their management responsibilities, they can enforce any interventions that are necessary by the interdisciplinary teams and ensure that interventions become the standard of care for high-fall-risk care recipients.
- *Nursing assistants and LPNs from acute care and extended care.* Nursing assistants and LPNs are generally the most affected by the interventions implemented by the fall team. These individuals can help educate their peers on the interventions and also act as fall reduction advocates by collecting data for the submission of aggregate reviews.
- *Pharmacist.* The pharmacist reviews medications of all high-fall-risk care recipients when they are identified and immediately after a fall. Pharmacists help to identify issues with medications and notify physicians when medications need to be adjusted. This is very important because many falls are the result of medication errors or adjustments to medicines.
- *Occupational therapist or physical therapist.* Occupational and physical therapists provide balance and strength assessments for high-fall-risk care recipients. These individuals can also assess the ability of a care recipient to use specific interventions, taking into account grip strength and other factors.
- *Physician/nurse practitioner.* The physician/nurse practitioner reviews the medical history and stability of the high-fall-risk care recipient when admitted and immediately after a fall. The physician/nurse practitioner should identify aspects of the medical history that could contribute to falls.

Nonclinical staff responsibilities should include the following:

- *Patient safety manager/quality management coordinator.* The patient safety manager or quality management coordinator can facilitate the team if there is no falls clinical specialist. This staff can also act as a liaison between the team and the management of the facility and provide data to the team to help determine the impact of the interventions taken.
- *Facility manager.* The facility manager can help to ensure that the environment of care is set up to reduce falls. He or she can train the janitorial staff to perform environmental assessments to remove clutter from rooms and ensure that spills are cleaned up promptly, among other responsibilities. The facility manager can also identify fall hazards related to cleaning supplies, such as a particular cleaning agent causing the floor to be sticky, and may assess the environment in common rooms to ensure that furniture is safe for those who are at a high risk of falls.
- *Supply procurement and distribution manager.* The supply procurement and distribution manager can help facilities purchase items that reduce the risk of falls and fall-related injuries, and can also ensure that supplies are adequate and the correct products are purchased.
- *Biotechnology manager.* The biotechnology manager can ensure that all devices are in working order to reduce the risk of care recipients falling and can also look into devices that were involved in falls, such as wheelchairs or walkers.
- *Transportation manager.* One facility added its transportation manager after several falls had occurred on transportation vans. Although this may not be useful in your facility, it is a good idea to add people to the team from areas other than patient or resident care if falls are occurring.

When to Do Assessments

Health care organizations traditionally include functional and nutritional assessments when evaluating newly admitted individuals. In many organizations, a fall risk assessment is conducted as part of the general admission assessment on all care recipients when they first enter the system or as it is triggered by certain responses or scoring levels on the functional screening. Elsewhere, however, fall assessment is performed only if and when a full-scale functional assessment is ordered, leaving an opportunity that may be as long as two days during which a vulnerable person could fall. If the data show that this is, in fact, happening, the organization needs to reexamine its protocol.[4]

Facility residents should be assessed for their risk of falling at several different junctures, according to Jacob Dimant, president of the American Medical Directors Association (AMDA). As noted in AMDA's Falls and Fall Risk Clinical Practice Guideline (CPG), "Sometimes, the actual fall is just the tip of the iceberg." Numerous risk factors are associated with care recipient falls, and an incomplete diagnosis of the reasons for a fall can result in repeat incidents. For example, a previous fall may have brought about a fear of falling, leading to reduced mobility, deconditioning, and loss of muscle strength and balance. A fall can also be the first visible sign of an acute illness such as pneumonia. In addition, neurological or cardiac illnesses, musculoskeletal problems, visual impairments, neuropathies, bowel or bladder incontinence, dehydration, and orthostatic hypotension brought on by medications all represent risk factors for falls.

It is critical, therefore, that a risk assessment be conducted upon admission, which is considered a time of high risk for the care recipient—especially if he or she is cognitively impaired. An older person's confusion can be magnified by a new, unfamiliar environment, which could put him or her at increased risk of a fall. Staff should conduct a quick assessment of the care recipient to identify any immediate risk factors.

According to the AMDA's Falls and Fall Risk CPG, a more comprehensive fall evaluation should then be performed within 7 to 14 days and incorporated into the care recipient's overall care plan. This assessment would, for example, gauge whether a care recipient has muscle weakness and gait problems. If so, rehabilitation can be instituted if the care recipient and family are willing. The comprehensive fall assessment should be revisited on a regular basis and repeated if a new fall occurs.

When a fall occurs, staff must immediately assess the injury, if any. If an injury is determined, it must be promptly treated. Staff should then make every attempt to identify the cause of the fall. Circumstances surrounding the fall are critical for diagnosing its cause, and many facilities generate a short-form checklist such as in Figure 3-1 on page 56, which prompts personnel to follow a prescribed process after a fall incident.

This is usually followed by a more comprehensive report, such as the Comprehensive Evaluation Postfall: Checklist 2 (*see* Figure 3-2, page 57). Dimant notes that causes of falls belong to one of two main categories: those inherent to the person and those that are environmental. Process indicators are, therefore, usually grouped according to category.

Individualized Care Plan

An organization's interdisciplinary team has the responsibility to evaluate each resident and to customize his or her care, integrating clinical and environmental interventions. If a resident with mobility problems is at risk of falling, one strategy might be to position the resident's bed in a low position or put it right on the floor.

FIGURE 3-1

Physical Assessment Following a Fall: Checklist 1

Name ______________________________ Date of fall ________________

Vital signs

Heart rate ______________

Heart rhythm regular ______________ irregular ____________

Blood pressure lying down ____________ standing ____________

Physical Exam

Active or independent range of motion:

Neck		yes _____	no_____			
Shoulders	Rt	yes _____	no_____	Lt	yes _____	no_____
Wrists	Rt	yes _____	no_____	Lt	yes _____	no_____
Hands	Rt	yes _____	no_____	Lt	yes _____	no_____
Hips	Rt	yes _____	no_____	Lt	yes _____	no_____
Knees	Rt	yes _____	no_____	Lt	yes _____	no_____
Ankles	Rt	yes _____	no_____	Lt	yes _____	no_____
Feet	Rt	yes _____	no_____	Lt	yes _____	no_____

Observations of Resident

Shortening and external rotation of lower extremities Rt ______ Lt_____

Swelling	Location ______________________________	
Redness/bruising	Location ______________________________	
Abrasions	Location ______________________________	
Pain on movement	Location ______________________________	
Shortness of breath	yes _____	no_____
Impaired balance	yes _____	no_____
Loss of consciousness	yes _____	no_____
Change in cognition	yes _____	no_____

Assessment of Environment

Dim lighting	yes _____	no_____
Glare	yes _____	no_____
Uneven flooring	yes _____	no_____
Wet or slippery floor	yes _____	no_____
Poor fit of seating device	yes _____	no_____
Inappropriate footwear	yes _____	no_____
Inappropriate eyewear	yes _____	no_____
Loose carpet or throw rugs	yes _____	no_____
Use of full-length side rails in bed	yes _____	no_____
Lack of hallway rails in area of fall	yes _____	no_____
Inappropriate assistive devices (fit or condition)	yes _____	no_____
Lack of grab bars in bathroom	yes _____	no_____
Cluttered areas	yes _____	no_____

Other environmental causes ______________________________

Source: Barbara Resnick, Ph.D., C.R.N.P., associate professor, University of Maryland School of Nursing, Baltimore.

FIGURE 3-2

Comprehensive Evaluation Postfall: Checklist 2

Name ______________________ Date of fall ______________

Underlying Medical Problems			
Orthostatic hypotension	yes _____	no _____	Management _____
Balance problems	yes _____	no _____	Management _____
Dizziness/vertigo	yes _____	no _____	Management _____
Other	yes _____	no _____	Management _____
Medications			
Diuretics	yes _____	no _____	Management _____
Cardiovascular meds	yes _____	no _____	Management _____
Antipsychotics	yes _____	no _____	Management _____
Antianxiety agents	yes _____	no _____	Management _____
Sleeping agents	yes _____	no _____	Management _____
Antidepressants	yes _____	no _____	Management _____
Functional Status			
Impaired sitting balance	yes _____	no _____	Management _____
Impaired standing balance	yes _____	no _____	Management _____
Independent ambulation	yes _____	no _____	Management _____
Independent toileting	yes _____	no _____	Management _____
Sensory Problems			
Evidence of impaired vision	yes _____	no _____	Management _____
Evidence of impaired sensation	yes _____	no _____	Management _____
Evidence of impaired hearing	yes _____	no _____	Management _____
Psychological Status			
Evidence of depression	yes _____	no _____	Management _____
Evidence of change in cognition	yes _____	no _____	Management _____
Evidence of impaired judgment	yes _____	no _____	Management _____

Action taken ______________________________

That way, if the resident falls, the risk of injury is minimized. However, other consequences must be considered when lowering the positioning of the bed. For instance, the team must determine how this position affects the resident's mobility and what effect this position has on staff members' ability to provide safe care.

In addition, the team can identify a fall risk reduction program that focuses on the population served. Strategies include taking the following actions:

- Install bed alarms or redesign bed alarm checks and tests.
- Install self-latching locks on utility rooms.
- Restrict window openings.
- Install alarms on exits.
- Add fall reduction to the education of care recipients and their families.
- Improve and standardize nurse call systems.
- Use "low beds" for those at risk for falls.
- Revise staffing procedures.
- Counsel individual caregivers.

Home care and long term care staff should look closely at the layout of the room. Staff should consider moving around the room, identifying vision impairments in order to detect anything that could pose a tripping hazard, such as carpet or furniture. Similarly, a behavioral health facility or unit may need to look more closely at the effects of various medications on the mobility of their client population.

Assistive devices such as canes, tripods, wheelchairs, and walkers can also help the resident to manipulate the environment and reduce the risk of falling. However, these devices must be in good repair, within easy reach, and available for the resident's use. "If the walker that the resident needs in order to get to the bathroom is stored in the corner, it won't do the resident any good," says Marianna Kern Grachek, executive director of long term care and assisted living accreditation at the Joint Commission.[5]

A fall team might create a fall reduction committee to assess new individuals or care recipients for fall potential; to regularly review falls, evaluate interventions, and look for trends and patterns; and to communicate its findings to other staff. Before full implementation of a fall risk assessment tool and as part of its ongoing research, a fall team might also choose to conduct a six-month pilot study on a general medical unit. With a fall risk assessment tool that uses care recipient indexes of falls—such as gait disturbance, confusion, previous falls, generalized weakness and incontinence—each fall could be given a numeric value based on the severity of the risk.[6]

Given the identified risk(s), the care recipient would then be assigned a fall risk score and be categorized as either a low risk or high risk for falling. Interventions can then be chosen by the caregiver from the fall risk assessment tool and become part of the care recipient's overall safety plan of care (*see* Figure 3-3, page 59).

The fall team could use the pilot study to adjust the numeric values on any determined risk factors. For example, if data showed that age was not a significant predictor of falls, whereas gait disturbance was, the fall risk assessment tool could assign a lesser numeric value to age and a higher numeric value to gait disturbance.

When implementing the fall risk assessment tool organizationwide, the fall team must make staff education a priority. In an inpatient setting, this might consist of unit-based in-services, posters, staff meetings, educational workshops, and/or an educational fair on fall risk assessment and fall reduction.

The fall risk assessment might also include a *root cause analysis* performed on each actual inpatient in order to expose possible relationships between assessed fall risks and root causes. A fall cause analysis tool is developed to gather information on individual care recipient fall risks, cause of fall, and fall outcomes immediately after each fall (*see* Figure 3-4, page 60). This tool is usually returned to the fall team's nursing leader, who enters the information in a database of analyzed care recipient falls.

The fall team can analyze these data to identify care recipient fall risks and their relationships to the fall root cause. For example, one health care organization found that approximately 80% of the care recipients who fell in its facility were confused, had gait disturbance, and were attempting to toilet alone. In performing additional analysis of the data, this organization's fall team began to distinguish trends among the three care recipient populations (medical, surgical, and psychiatric). Care recipients with surgical diagnoses were more likely to fall during the middle or later part of their hospitalization, whereas care recipients with medical diagnoses tended to fall soon after the day of admission.

FIGURE 3-3

Fall Risk Assessment Tool

FALL RISK ASSESSMENT

- ❑ Gait disturbance (shuffling, jerking, swaying) **(4)**
- ❑ Dizziness / syncope in an upright position **(3)**
- ❑ Confused all the time **(3)**
- ❑ Nocturia / Incontinent **(3)**
- ❑ Intermittent confusion **(2)**
- ❑ Generalized weakness **(2)**
- ❑ "High risk" drugs (diuretics, narcotics, sedatives, Anti-psychotics, substance abuse withdrawal) **(2)**
- ❑ Previous falls w/n last 12 months **(2)**
- ❑ Osteoporosis **(1)**
- ❑ Hearing and / or visually impaired **(1)**
- ❑ 70 years old or greater **(1)**

A score of 1–3 points indicates a LOW RISK for falling.

- ✓ **Reassess fall risks Q 12 hours**
- ✓ **Give patient/family fall education brochure**

A score of 4 points or more indicates a HIGH RISK for falling.

- ✓ **Implement ALL interventions below, as appropriate:**

1- Apply neon pink bracelet to patient; apply neon pink name card to door
2- Communicate patient's fall risks to interdisciplinary team members
3- Communicate patient's fall risks to patient/family →*give fall education brochure*
4- **Encourage family participation in patient safety**
5- Offer frequent toileting
6- Environmental safety: avoid clutter in room, keep call bell and telephone near, leave door open, use a night light, top 2 side rails up
7- Do not leave unattended on bedside commode or toilet
8- Use nonslip socks (order from CDS) or shoes
9- Consult:
Decentralized Pharmacist for possible medication interactions
Physical Therapy for new mobility or ADL problems (MD order required)
10- Use diversionary activities (diversion box) to prevent wandering
11- Order walker from CDS to assist with stability/walking
12- Up in wheelchair at desk or hall for observation
13- Obtain a sitter →notify Nursing Administration (MD order required)
14- Use a soft belt or roll belt (initiate restraint procedure as well)
15- Other safety interventions

ADMISSION Fall Risk Score: ____________
Interventions (circle) 1-7, 8, 9, 10, 11, 12, 13, 14, 15
other__________________________
Name/Title______________________________

FIGURE 3-4

Fall Cause Analysis Tool

Fall Cause Analysis
(To be completed after a fall occurs)

Fall Date:_____________ Fall Time:_______________ Patient ID:_____________
Location of Fall:_____________ Age:_______ Gender:_______
Primary Diagnosis: (circle one) *Medical* *Surgical* *Psychiatric*

Check the following fall risk factors present at time of fall:

- ☐ Generalized weakness
- ☐ Gait disturbance
- ☐ Confused
- ☐ Attempting to toilet alone
- ☐ Previous fall in last 12 months
- ☐ Dizziness/syncope
- ☐ High risk drugs (diuretics, narcotics, sedatives, antipsychotics)
- ☐ Patient alone at time of fall
- ☐ History of CVA/TIA
- ☐ Dizziness/syncope
- ☐ Incontinent

Check the following fall prevention interventions used at time of fall:

- ☐ On Fall Protocol at time of fall
  - ○ Score: High Low
- ☐ Family at bedside
- ☐ Non-slip socks/shoes in use
- ☐ Frequent toileting offered
- ☐ Assistive device (walker, cane, adult walking device)
- ☐ Patient room/floor free of clutter
- ☐ Call bell in reach, telephone in reach
- ☐ Bed in low position

Fall Outcome(s):

- ☐ No injury
- ☐ Abrasion
- ☐ Laceration
- ☐ Fracture minor major
- ☐ Contusion
- ☐ Placed on Fall Protocol
- ☐ Transferred to ICU
- ☐ Restraints applied
- ☐ MD Assessment done

Through root causes analysis, a fall team is able to determine fall risks and their relationships to fall root causes in a retrospective manner. The team is also better equipped to take effective action as part of its fall reduction program.

SIDEBAR 3-1

Ongoing Older Adult Fall Risk Evaluation

1. All older persons who are under the care of a health professional (or their caregivers) should be asked at least once a year about falls.
2. All older persons who report a single fall should be observed as they stand up from a chair without using their arms, walk several paces, and return (for example, the "Get Up & Go Test"). Those demonstrating no difficulty or unsteadiness need no further assessment.
3. Persons who have difficulty or demonstrate unsteadiness performing this test require further assessment.

Staff Education

When ensuring and maintaining a successful risk assessment process, all staff must be educated about the physiology of falls, about fall risk factors, and about specific care recipients at risk for falling.

Staff competence in keeping care recipients safe from falls while performing such tasks as transfers and bathing should be assessed through return demonstrations. Written posttests or verbal repetition of education might be more appropriate in other instances. For example, housekeepers who have received training in what to do if they walk past a care recipient's room and notice that the care recipient is about to fall out of bed can be asked to describe how they would handle the situation. "Competence assessment must be individually determined based on an employee's position," according to Christian. "However, all staff members are responsible for helping to ensure patient safety."

In approaching risk assessment, it is important that caregivers keep in mind specific assessment recommendations regarding those who have previously experienced a fall and those who may be at risk of falling.

SIDEBAR 3-2

Ongoing Fall Risk Evaluation for Older Adults at Risk

1. Older persons who present for medical attention because of a fall, report recurrent falls in the past year, or demonstrate abnormalities of gait and/or balance should have a fall evaluation performed. This evaluation should be performed by a clinician with appropriate skills and experience, which may necessitate referral to a specialist (for example, geriatrician).
2. A fall evaluation is defined as an assessment that includes a history of fall circumstances, medications, acute or chronic medical problems, and mobility levels; an examination of vision, gait and balance, and lower extremity joint function; an examination of basic neurological function, including mental status, muscle strength, lower extremity peripheral nerves, proprioception, reflexes, tests of cortical, extrapyramidal, and cerebellar function; and assessment of basic cardiovascular status, including heart rate and rhythm, postural pulse and blood pressure, and, if appropriate, heart rate and blood pressure responses to carotid sinus stimulation.[7]

Strokes as a Risk Factor

In preparing interventions that combat the causes of care recipient falls, it is important that staff be educated on how to identify care recipients who are particularly prone to falls. For example, strokes are one of the primary risk factors for care recipient falls. In acute care centers and various rehabilitation processes, stroke patients are reportedly more prone to falls than other care recipient populations.[8–10]

In one case-control study, stroke was proven to be a risk factor for hip fracture among women. The same study identified previous strokes as a factor in a sample of femoral neck-fracture care recipients[11,12] and showed that the reported percentages of stroke care recipients suffering falls during their hospitalization included 14% in acute care,[13] 24% in a rehabilitation setting, and 39% in geriatric rehabilitation.[14]

Another report, "Risk Factors for Falls of Hospitalized Stroke Patients," by J.A. Tutuarimia, R.N., J.H.P.; A. van Straten, M.Sc.; M. Limburg, M.D., Ph.D., and others, studied a cohort of 720 stroke patients (346 women and 374 men with a median age of 75 years) from 23 hospitals in the Netherlands to assess the fall incidence and risk factors for patients hospitalized as the result of an acute stroke.[15]

This study focused on patients with confirmed stroke that lasted greater than 24 hours or led to death. The data, abstracted from the medical and nursing records, showed 77% of the patients had suffered a cerebral infarct, 17% had suffered a hemorrhage, and 6% had suffered an undefined stroke. There was a total of 173 falls, and the study recorded 104 patients, or 14%, who fell at least once. The incidence of falls was 8.9 per 1,000 patients per day. The daily incidence was 6.2 per 1,000 patients for first falls and 17.9 per 1,000 patients for second falls. Heart disease, mental decline, and urinary incontinence were incremental risk factors for first falls, whereas the use of major psychotropic drugs lowered the fall risk. Most falls occurred during the day. Approximately 25% of the falls caused slight-to-severe injury, whereas three falls, or 2%, led to hip fractures. The study concluded that identification of patients at risk is a likely first step toward the implementation of fall reduction measures for patients.

With falls being recognized as a common occurrence in stroke patients, it has been assumed that injuries and other consequences of falls often have a negative effect on the rehabilitation process and its outcome. For example, restricted activity as a result of the fear of new falls can impede the rehabilitation process. In looking at the predictors of falls, researchers have found that the number of hospital falls among stroke patients correlates with this group's risk of falls after discharge from the hospital. Those with previous falls have shown lower activity levels and depressed moods, which, coupled with other factors, can lead to added pressure on their caregivers.[16]

Among the conclusions in a multifactorial case-control study was the finding that a history of falls, impaired decision-making ability, restlessness, generalized weakness, and abnormal hematocrit level were independent fall risk factors among stroke patients in acute care.[17]

Multiple Risk Factors

Several studies have shown that the risk of falling increases dramatically as the number of risk factors increase. One such study surveyed community-dwelling elderly persons and reported that the percentage of persons falling increased from 27% for those with no or one risk factor to 78% for those with four or more risk factors. Another study reported that the

SIDEBAR 3-3

Fall Risk Factors as Assessment Elements

Assessments should identify conditions that may increase fall risk.

Demographic and History
- Patient's age
- Patient's sex
- History of previous falls
- Fear of falling
- Length of stay in the health care facility

Diagnosis or Conditions
- Cardiac arrhythmias
- Transient ischemic attacks
- Stroke
- Parkinson's disease
- Delirium
- Dementia illnesses
- Depression
- Musculoskeletal conditions such as myopathy and deformities
- Problems with mobility/gait
- Lower-extremity strength
- History of fractures
- Ambulatory aids
- Orthostatic hypotension
- Elimination status (for example, incontinence of bowel or bladder)
- Visual and auditory impairments
- Dizziness
- Dehydration
- Other acute and subacute medical illnesses

Medications
- Diuretics
- Analgesics
- Hypnotics/tranquilizers
- Laxatives/cathartics
- Polypharmacy (multiple medications)

Environmental and Other
- Use of restraints
- Intravenous therapy/heparin lock
- Footwear
- Confined to a chair
- Post-op

percentage of community-living persons with recurrent falls increased from 10% to 69% as the number of risk factors increased from one to four or more.[18,19]

Others believe that of greater importance than the independent effect of each factor alone is the combination of multiple risk factors, concurrently present and compounding the contribution of each factor to the risk of falls.[20] In identifying risk factors, then, it is important that staff appreciate the interaction and probable synergism between multiple risk factors.

An example of this "cycle" of risk factors is the care recipient with a fear of falling. Persons who fall and are worried about falling again, it has been shown, are more likely to show declines in gait and balance over a two-year follow-up than fallers who were not worried about falling again,[21] and low fall-related self-efficacy has been associated with a decline in a person's ability to perform active daily living.[22] Because the direct association between falls and fear of falling has not been clearly drawn, any of the following could explain their relationship: Falls may cause fear of falling, fear of falling may cause falls, and the two outcomes may be related to shared risk factors and not themselves causally related.[23] If falls lead to falling and vice versa, then development of one may start a cascade effect, with a resulting escalation of risk for functional decline and other adverse outcomes. Furthermore, if these syndromes have shared risk factors, then individuals with these characteristics would be at particularly high risk of developing this cycle, and this group would be important to target for reduction strategies to reduce falls and fear of falling.

As a consequence of multiple risk factors and their contribution to care recipient falls, a number of scoring systems have been developed in which the numbers of present risk factors are added together by means of different algorithms to reflect the fall risk.[24–26] These systems are discussed later in this chapter.

Staff Communication

High-quality communication among staff during shift changes or nursing unit transfers is also critical. Changes in a care recipient's behavior or condition from one shift to the next may signal increased risk for falls and the need for a care plan revision. Ideally, communications should be both written and verbal. Thorough documentation in the clinical record provides vital information for all caregivers.

Thorough communication among all care team members helps to ensure that care is provided in a coordinated manner. "Everyone who provides care to an individual may hold a piece of the puzzle that, and when fit into the whole, will reduce fall risk for that care recipient," suggests Joint Commission surveyor Vicki Christian. Proactive interdisciplinary conferences provide an opportunity for each staff member to offer suggestions about how to reduce falls. "If a care recipient falls, the team should meet promptly to identify strategies to reduce the risk of future falls with this care recipient and others," says Christian.

Communication and transfer of information between and among health care professionals are essential to reducing fall risk. Coordinated communication can help staff to revise care plans appropriately and implement proactive fall reduction strategies.

Leaders should create and nurture a culture that values open and direct communication among staff and between caregivers, care recipients, and care recipient families. All communication, regardless of the position and the rank of the communicator, must be valued. All caregivers must be expected to communicate information vital to the provision of coordinated and collaborative care.

Communication with family members is also critical to thorough assessment of fall risk. Staff should inform family members about factors that increase fall risk and inquire about the presence of any such factors. Educating the care recipient and family about fall reduction strategies can help reduce fall risk in the health care organization *and* after the individual is discharged. Techniques to improve strength and balance are particularly important.

Attentive and thoughtful communication can also serve as avoidance. Before a staff member leaves a care recipient's room, the most important words he or she can utter are "Is there anything else I can do for you before I leave?" "This seems so simple," Christian says, "but it reminds the care recipient to ask for help with tasks that might result in a fall if done by the care recipient on his or her own."

Medication

Medication assessments and reassessments must

take into account all prescription and over-the-counter drugs and supplements the individual is taking, medication allergies, and history of substance abuse—including the use of tranquilizers or other prescription drugs.

In doing the initial assessment, it is wise to get the medical history from someone who really knows the care recipient. "Many times, the children of a geriatric care recipient live out of state and don't really know what's going on in the home," says Joint Commission surveyor Anne Piper. "A husband or wife may bias the information to make the spouse look better. A person who knows how the care recipient functions in performing the activities of daily living is the best source of information. If the information seems questionable," Piper advises, "you need to consider doing a reassessment and more closely monitor the individual. In any event, the reliability of the history should be factored into the assessment."

Even when the original information is sound, low-risk individuals can quickly become high-risk if, for example, there is a change in medications or in their ability to perform daily living activities. For this reason, many effective assessment tools call for the information to be validated in 24 hours.

Categorizing Risk Assessment Tools

According to recent data, the fall rates in nursing homes and hospitals are approximately three times that of falls among the community-dwelling elderly over age 65.[27] With the potential for serious injury when a long term care resident falls, the Centers for Medicare & Medicaid Services mandates the reporting of all fall incidents. Marking the fall indicator on the quarterly minimum data set triggers a resident assessment protocol, which necessitates a fuller investigation of the cause of the incident.

Yet, as illustrated in the previous fall example of the 42-year-old man with alcoholic cirrhosis, when it comes to fall assessment, the act of fulfilling regulatory requirements is only a small part of the process.

Some experts have categorized fall risk assessment tools based on their setting and discipline. As outlined in the report "Assessing the Risk of Falls: Guidelines for Selecting Appropriate Measures for Clinical Practice Settings,"[28] by Karen L. Perell, it is the setting and discipline that often determine which assessment tools will be most conducive and most effective. The three categories are (1) comprehensive medical assessments performed by geriatricians or nurse practitioners in nursing homes or outpatient settings, (2) nursing fall risk assessments performed in hospitals and nursing homes, and (3) functional mobility assessments completed by physical therapists or physicians in an outpatient setting.

Geriatricians and nurse practitioners generally use the comprehensive medical assessment to evaluate and treat care recipients at risk for falls or care recipients who have recently fallen.[29] A comprehensive medical assessment entails in-depth medical evaluation of fall risk factors specific to the care recipient, such as the care recipient's psychological status, mobility dysfunction, history of falls, elimination frequency, acute and chronic illnesses, and sensory deficits.[30] The assessment can be part of an overall geriatric assessment or part of a postfall assessment that focuses on identifying fall risk factors that can be treated to reduce the likelihood of a fall.[29] As mentioned previously, the likelihood of a fall increases or decreases according to the number of risk factors.[31] Such an assessment can be time consuming and often requires a team of physicians.[32]

The nursing assessment has been widely performed in hospitals and nursing homes. It typically employs specific screening instruments or forms, such as the Morse Fall Scale, the STRATIFY model,[33] and the Hendrich Fall Risk Model,[34] to identify who is likely to fall based on intrinsic, or specific-related, fall risk factors. These instruments are most widely used by nursing staff at the time of the care recipient's admission to a hospital or long term care facility. They are also periodically updated per shift, daily, or weekly, depending on the care recipient's condition. They tend to be short and do not require intensive assessment of the care recipient. Poor scores on this assessment tool often trigger either further assessment or nursing intervention aimed at reducing the care recipient's risk.[35]

As Perell's report points out, it is quite common for an individual hospital or long term care facility to rely on fall risk factors from the literature or retrospective chart reviews of its own care recipients' falls in developing its own nursing fall risk assessment scale.

Functional assessment instruments identify gait and balance deficits, which rank high among the risk factors that pose the highest relative risk for the elderly who fall. Only muscle weakness—a contributing factor to gait and balance deficits—and history of falls rank higher. Consequently, functional assessment instruments are commonly used to assess falls among community-dwelling older people.

These instruments—the Tinetti Performance Oriented Mobility Assessment, the Dynamic Gait Index,[36] and the Timed Get Up & Go Test[37] among others—focus on functional limitations in gait and balance. Physical therapists are the most frequent users of functional assessment tools for community-dwelling care recipients, most often on an outpatient basis, regardless of medical diagnosis. Some geriatricians use functional assessments as part of a comprehensive geriatric assessment. In clinical settings, poor scores typically trigger interventions to improve function, such as muscle strengthening, gait and balance training, or aerobic exercise.[38]

Choosing the Appropriate Assessment Tool

There is no one right assessment tool for all organizations or all populations, but choosing the best fit for an organization can make the difference in reducing falls.

The comprehensive medical assessment mentioned above provides valuable clinical information, according to Perell, but because of its length and scope it may not be an appropriate initial assessment tool. The comprehensive medical assessment is more fitting and more effective as a secondary assessment for high-risk care recipients who have been identified as such by nurse staff and functional mobility assessments. It is the nursing staff and functional mobility assessments that provide quick, reliable, and valid information in identifying high-risk care recipients for further fall-related assessments and appropriate interventions.

Perell notes that in choosing from the multitude of nursing staff and functional mobility assessments, "It is important to choose tools that have been subjected to psychometric testing; that have been developed or studied with a similar care recipient population; that have written procedures explicitly outlining appropriate use of the tool; that have a scale that can be administered in a reasonable amount of time; and that denote established thresholds indicating when to initiate interventions."[39]

While these criteria apply regardless of setting, the specific instrument chosen might vary, depending on the setting and types of professionals responsible for performing the assessments. Different types of setting—acute care, outpatient, extended care—require use of different assessment scales.

There is a great variety of adequate screening tools already being used, measured, and improved in existing fall reduction programs. Although many health care organizations continue to initiate their own assessment programs, it is important to consider and incorporate existing models in their development process.

One model that has been commonly adapted by health care organizations is the Morse Risk Assessment Tool. Developed by Janice M. Morse after a 10-year period of following detailed background research into risk factors associated with falling, it is one of the few available assessment tools designed for use in an acute care environment. Results from definitive tests performed to ensure accuracy, reliability, and sensitivity have shown that the tool has a strong validity and sensitivity.[40]

According to Morse, because multifactorial etiologic factors of care recipient falls should be at the core of all fall reduction programs, risk assessment tools serve as the impetus to successful intervention strategies. Siding with the more all-encompassing classification that categorizes falls as *accidental, unanticipated physiologic, or anticipated physiologic,*[41] Morse contends that fall interventions must be linked to each etiologic factor. Morse views the inclusive nature of her classification as an appropriate fit with approaches to reduction, one that helps determine basic intervention principles for fall reduction programs. Beginning with a review of this classification, an adapted version of her report on the elements of a strong fall reduction program is illustrated in Figure 3-5.

Like many other models, the Morse tool insists that assessment of risk should be performed on admission and that frequent reassessment should occur throughout the hos-

FIGURE 3-5

Morse Report on Fall Reduction Programs

Accidental falls occur when care recipients fall unintentionally (for example, they may trip, slip, or fall because of a failure of equipment). Although approximately 14% of all falls are accidental, most fall reduction strategies are targeted toward this type of fall. It is important to recognize that care recipients who experience an accidental fall cannot be identified before the fall and do not score at risk of falling on a predictive instrument, such as the Morse Fall Scale (MFS). The MFS is a quick, easy method of determining the risk of falling. It consists of six items and has established reliability and validity testing.

Unanticipated physiologic falls occur when the physical causes of the falls are not reflected in the care recipients' risk factors for falls. These falls are caused by physical conditions that cannot be predicted until the care recipient falls. For example, the fall may be due to fainting, a seizure, or a pathologic fracture of the hip. Unanticipated physiologic falls constitute 8% of all falls in a hospital setting.

Anticipated physiologic falls occur with care recipients whose score on the MFS indicates that they are at risk of falling. According to the scale, these care recipients have some of the following characteristics: a prior fall, weak or impaired gait, use of a walking aid, intravenous

(continued)

FIGURE 3-5 (continued)

access, or impaired mental status. These care recipients are expected to fall. Even if the actual "trigger" for the fall may be that a care recipient with an impaired gait tripped because of the impaired gait, it is expected that the care recipient will trip; therefore, the cause of the fall is classified as anticipated rather than accidental. Anticipated physiologic falls constitute 78% of all falls in the hospital population.

The MFS is a rapid and simple method of assessing a care recipient's likelihood of falling. A large majority of nurses, approximately 82.9%, rate the scale as "quick and easy to use," and 54% estimate that it takes less than 3 minutes to rate a care recipient. It consists of six variables that are quick and easy to score, and it has been shown to have predictive validity and interrater reliability. The MFS is used widely in acute care settings, both in hospital and long term care inpatient settings.

Morse Fall Scale

Item	Scale	Scoring
1. History of falling; immediate or within 3 months	No 0 Yes 25	_____ _____
2. Secondary diagnosis	No 0 Yes 15	_____ _____
3. Ambulatory aid Bed rest/nurse assist Crutches/cane/walker Furniture	 0 15 30	_____
4. IV/heparin lock	No 0 Yes 25	_____ _____
5. Gait/transferring Normal/bed rest/immobile Weak Impaired	 0 15 30	_____
6. Mental status Oriented to own ability Forgets limitations	 0 15	_____

The items in the scale are scored as follows:

History of falling. This is scored as 25 if the care recipient has fallen during the present hospital admission, or if there is an immediate history of physiologic falls, such as from seizures or an impaired gait prior to admission. If the care recipient has not fallen, this is scored 0. Note: If a care recipient falls for the first time, then his or her score immediately increases by 25.

(continued)

FIGURE 3-5 (continued)

Secondary diagnosis. This is scored as 15 if more than one medical diagnosis is listed on the care recipient's chart; if not, score 0.

Ambulatory aids. This is scored as 0 if the care recipient walks without a walking aid (even if assisted by a nurse), uses a wheelchair, or is on bed rest and does not get out of bed at all. If the care recipient uses crutches, a cane, or a walker, this item scores 15; if the care recipient ambulates clutching onto the furniture for support, score this item 30.

Intravenous therapy. This is scored as 20 if the care recipient has an intravenous apparatus or a heparin lock inserted; if not, score 0.

Gait. A normal gait is characterized by the care recipient walking with head erect, arms swinging freely at the side, and striding without hesitation. This gait scores 0. With a weak gait (score as 10), the care recipient is stooped but is able to lift the head while walking without losing balance. Steps are short and the care recipient may shuffle. With an impaired gait (score 20), the care recipient may have difficulty rising from a chair—attempting to get up by pushing on the arms of the chair or by bouncing (for example, by using several attempts to rise). The care recipient's head is down, and he or she watches the ground. Because the care recipient's balance is poor, he or she grasps the furniture, a support person, or a walking aid for support and cannot walk without this assistance.

Mental status. When using this scale, mental status is measured by checking the care recipient's own self-assessment of his or her ability to ambulate. Ask the care recipient, "Are you able to go the bathroom alone or do you need assistance?" If the care recipient's reply judging his or her own ability is consistent with the ambulatory order, the care recipient is rated as "normal" and scored 0. If the care recipient's response is not consistent with the nursing orders or if the care recipient's response is unrealistic, then the care recipient is considered to overestimate his or her own abilities and to be forgetful of limitations, and scored as 15.

Scoring and risk level. The score is then tallied and recorded on the care recipient's chart. Risk level and recommended actions (for example, no interventions needed, standard fall interventions, high-risk interventions) are then identified.

Note: The MFS should be calibrated for each particular health care setting or unit so that strategies are targeted to those most at risk. In other words, risk cutoff scores may be different, depending on if you are using it in an acute care hospital, nursing home, or rehabilitation facility. In addition, scales may be set differently between particular units within a given facility.

Sample Risk Level

Risk Level	MFS Score	Action
No Risk	0–24	Good basic nursing care
Low Risk	25–50	Implement standard fall interventions
High Risk	≥51	Implement high-risk fall interventions

Source: Morse J.M.: Preventing Patient Falls. Thousand Oaks, CA: Sage Publications, 1997. Adapted with permission.

pital stay. Many health care organizations have adapted the Morse tool to fit their setting and purpose.

A System for Strokes

Although scoring systems like the Morse scale offer strong content validity for use in general populations of the elderly, none of them are specifically intended for use in stroke patient populations. As mentioned previously, stroke patients are particularly susceptible to falls.

According to a report titled "Fall Prediction Index for Patients in Stroke Rehabilitation," by Lars Nyberg, R.P.T., Ph.D., and Yngve Gustafson, M.D., D.M.Sc.,[42] when tested in a geriatric stroke rehabilitation setting, the prediction accuracy of the Downton Index proved to be moderate. "It was concluded that adjustments to the index would be preferable if it was to be used in a population of stroke care recipients," the study reports. "The Fall Assessment Questionnaire (FAQ) showed rather high correlation with falls among male right-hemisphere stroke care recipients in rehabilitation, but that was in combination with a measure of behavioral impulsivity, which requires a rather complex instrumental setting, thus reducing its clinical usefulness."

The purpose of the Nyberg and Gustafson prospective investigation was, therefore, to develop an easily administered instrument for the identification of fall-prone individuals in stroke rehabilitation. An adapted version of this report is illustrated in Example 3-1.

Measuring the Progress of Risk Assessment

Depending on the population, risk assessment

EXAMPLE 3-1

Fall Prediction Index for Patients in Stroke Rehabilitation

Setting and Care Recipients

This study was performed at the stroke rehabilitation unit of the geriatric clinic at Umeå University Hospital, Sweden. Patients admitted to this 24-bed ward are the most severely affected third of the survivors of those admitted to the hospital for acute-phase stroke in the catchment area of Umeå University Hospital. These patients all need further rehabilitation and hospital stay after the acute phase and are transferred from acute care clinics, usually two to four weeks after the stroke.

All patients, numbering 142, admitted to rehabilitation after cerebrovascular accidents or other clinically similar conditions from November 1, 1991, through October 31, 1992, were included. Seven patients who were completely immobile and bedridden throughout their entire stay and who made no locomotion efforts were subsequently excluded from analysis because they were judged not to be at risk of falls, and rehabilitation was not possible. Thus, 135 patients remained, and their basic characteristics are summarized in Table 1.

The study was approved by the ethics committee of the Faculty of Medicine of Umeå University, and all subjects or their relatives gave their informed consent.

(continued)

EXAMPLE 3-1 (continued)

Table 1. Sample Characteristics at Inclusion in Study

Characteristic	
Mean±SD age, y	74.8±8.9
Sex, M/F	69/66
Diagnoses, n	
Nonembolic cerebral infarctions	74
Embolic cerebral infarctions	18
Cerebral infarctions, unspecified	10
Cerebral hemorrhages	19
Subarachnoid/subdural hemorrhages	5
Brain tumors (operated on)	4
Traumatic brain injuries	3
Brain abscesses (operated on)	2
Clinical signs, n	
Dysphasia	52
Dyspraxia	45
Visuospatial hemineglect	63
Median Katz ADL score (1st, 3rd quartiles)[1]	F (C, F)
Median MMSE score (1st, 3rd quartiles)[2]	20 (7, 27)

ADL indicates activities of daily living; MMSE, Mini-Mental State Examination.

1. Katz S., Ford A.B., et al.: Studies of illness in the aged. The index of ADL: a standardized measure of biological and psychosocial function. *J Am Med Assoc.* 1963;185:914–919.
2. Folstein M.F., Folstein S.E., et al.: "Mini-Mental State": a practical method for grading the cognitive state of patients for the clinician. *J Psychiatr Res.* 1975;12:189–198.

Assessments

Data on patient characteristics were collected during the first week of hospitalization at the geriatric rehabilitation unit. The stroke diagnoses were based on clinical examination and CT scan in accordance with the procedures of the Stroke Unit of Umeå University Hospital, the criteria of which have been published previously. The history of previous strokes and falls was taken from medical records, from the subjects themselves during admission interviews, or from their family members or caregivers. During the admission assessment, a physician recorded visual and hearing impairments if the subject was unable to read a short text in 10 mm block letters at reading distance or comprehend a conversation in a normal voice from a distance of 1 m. Clinical findings from the admission assessments and from the following one-week inclusion period were used when concurrent medical disorders and comorbidity were rated by means of standard clinical procedures.

A score of 7 or lower of a maximum of 9 on the Line Bisection Test was taken to indicate

(continued)

EXAMPLE 3-1 (continued)

visuospatial hemineglect. However, only 74% of the patients could complete this test. Dyspractic behavior and dysphasia, as well as visuospatial hemineglect for those who were not able to complete the Line Bisection Test, were estimated in multidisciplinary rehabilitation team consensus after comprehensive admission assessments and observations of the patients' behavior in activities performed during the inclusion period.

The location of brain lesions was determined by means of CT scan examinations and categorized: no lesions observed; right, left, or bilateral hemisphere cortical lesions; cerebellar lesions; mid-brain/brain-stem lesions; findings of bilateral white matter lesions (leukoaraiosis and multiple lacunar infarcts); and other (such as hydrocephalus).

Blood component analyses included erythrocyte sedimentation rate; white cell count; blood glucose and hemoglobin levels; and serum sodium, potassium, calcium, albumin, and creatinine levels. Venous blood samples were taken from the subjects in a fasting state and were part of the clinical routines used in this particular setting. Component values were rated as high, normal, or low, depending on how they related to the reference values used by the clinical chemistry laboratory contracted.

The performance of activities of daily living (ADL) was assessed according to the Katz Index, which includes six items: bathing, dressing, toileting, transferring, urinary continence, and feeding. The score ranges from A (independent in all items) to G (completely dependent). Ratings indicating dependence in the urinary continence item were taken to correspond to urinary incontinence.

Cognitive state was examined with the Mini-Mental State Examination (MMSE), including assessments of orientation, registration, attention, calculation, recall, language, and copying. The score ranges from 0 to 30, and a score of 23 points or less is usually considered to indicate cognitive impairment.

Motor function and postural stability were assessed by means of the Brunnström–Fugl-Meyer assessment scale. The motor function score ranges from 0 to 100, where 0 to 49 is graded as severe motor impairment, 50 to 84 as marked, 85 to 95 as moderate, and 96 to 100 as no or slight impairment. Motor function was assessed on both sides, but only the score of the most impaired side was used in the analysis of its relation to the fall risk. Furthermore, if the motor function scores of both sides were 95 or less, subjects were rated as bilaterally impaired. From a practical point of view, this cutoff score corresponds to findings of marked tendon reflex abnormalities or signs of marked dyscoordination in finger-nose and heel-knee coordination tests. The postural stability score, ranging from 0 to 14, includes assessments of postural stability and balance reactions in a sitting position, as well as bipedal and unipedal stance stability. A cutoff score of 9 or less corresponds to severe postural instability (for example, inability to stand steadily on both feet for one minute) or difficulties with one-legged stance in combination with reduced balance reactions in a sitting position.

Postural hypotension was defined as a drop of more than 10 mm Hg in systolic blood pressure

(continued)

EXAMPLE 3-1 (continued)

when a subject rises to a sitting position after a five-minute rest in a supine position. Medication data were abstracted from medical records and included only drugs prescribed for regular use. The groupings used were those suggested by Downton.

Falls

The patients were studied for 8 weeks (56 days) from their admission to the geriatric rehabilitation unit up to their discharge or death. They were thus studied for a median of 49 days, ranging from 3 to 56 days, with an interquartile range of 22 to 56 days. Falls were defined as incidents when the subject, due to an unexpected loss of balance, came to rest on the floor or an object below knee height. All such incidents that took place during the study period and that came to the knowledge of the nursing staff were reported on special fall-report forms. The incidence, characteristics, and injury consequences of these falls have been presented previously.

Statistical Analyses

Because of the wide range of the observation periods, survival analysis methods were used, describing the fall risk (dependent variable) as a function of time. For each subject, the time from admission to the first fall (for example, the event-free period) was calculated. If no falls occurred during the study period, observations were censored either at the end point of study (8 weeks) or on discharge or death. Univariate and multiple Cox regression analyses were used to assess the associations of patient-characteristic variables to the dependent variable. Variables associated with the fall risk by a value of $P < .10$ in the univariate analyses were selected for further analysis and tried in the multiple Cox regression modeling. The selection of the final model variables was based on three prerequisites: The inclusion of them should contribute significantly to the model (a significant change to the log-likelihood 2), they should be easy to rate in a clinical situation, and they should offer good content validity. The final Cox regression model was transformed into an index, by means of which the scores of the variables included were added together. Finally, the fit of the resulting index to the outcome variable was assessed with Cox regression and Kaplan-Meier analysis with log-rank test for statistical significance. SYSTAT and SPSS statistical software programs were used for the computation.

Results

During the first 8 weeks of rehabilitation, 49, or 36%, of the patients fell at least once, and 30, or 22%, fell twice or more. Table 2 on page 74 shows the univariate association of selected patient-characteristic variables with the fall risk. Variables selected for further multiple analyses (values of $P < .10$) included sex, signs of visuospatial neglect and dyspraxia, CT findings of bilateral hemispheric cortical or white matter lesions, Katz ADL score of E or lower, urinary incontinence, cognitive impairment (MMSE score < 24), bilateral motor impairment, severe postural stability impairment (score < 10), high blood glucose level, high white blood cell count, and the combined variable of use of any of the medication groups of diuretics, antidepressants, or sedatives. The dichotomous transformations of the functional scores were selected; because of clear threshold effects, they appeared to produce a stronger association with the dependent variable than their scale origins did.

(continued)

EXAMPLE 3-1 (continued)

Table 2. Univariate Cox Regression Analyses of Associations Between Patient Admission Characteristics and Fall Risk During Inpatient Stroke Rehabilitation

Variable	OR (95% CI)
Age, y	1.01 (0.98-1.04)
Male sex	2.08 (1.16-3.73)
Previous stroke diagnosis	1.26 (0.71-2.21)
Previous falls	1.19 (0.64-2.20)
Clinical signs	
Visual impairment	1.42 (0.80-2.51)
Hearing impairment	0.72 (0.32-1.60)
Dyspraxia	1.96 (1.10-3.47)
Visuospatial hemineglect	2.16 (1.20-3.90)
Dysphasia	1.36 (0.77-2.41)
Delirium	1.58 (0.76-3.28)
Depression	0.56 (0.20-1.56)
Urinary tract infection	0.99 (0.52-1.87)
Bilateral brain lesions including leukoaraiosis (CT)	2.03 (1.15-3.58)
High blood glucose level	2.13 (1.19-3.82)
High white blood cell count	1.87 (1.04-3.37)
Katz ADL score, A-G[1]	1.38 (1.12-1.71)
Katz ADL score, E or lower[1]	6.43 (1.99-20.71)
Urinary incontinence (Katz categorization[1])	4.05 (1.72-9.52)
MMSE score, 0-30[2]	0.98 (0.95-1.00)
Cognitively impaired (MMSE score <24[2])	2.26 (1.13-4.55)
Motor function score, 0-100[3]	1.00 (0.99-1.01)
Bilateral motor impairment (motor function score <96 on both sides)[3]	3.64 (1.31-10.14)
Postural stability score, 0-14[3]	0.92 (0.85-1.01)
Severe postural impairment (score <10)[3]	3.85 (1.38-10.72)
Orthostatic hypotension (>10 mm Hg drop in systolic blood pressure from supine to sitting)	1.37 (0.70-2.68)
Use of	
Diuretics	1.20 (0.67-2.12)
Antihypertensives other than diuretics	1.02 (0.57-1.85)
Laxatives	1.02 (0.58-1.79)
Antidepressants	1.49 (0.70-3.19)
Sedatives	1.06 (0.55-2.04)
Diuretics, antidepressants, or sedatives	1.62 (0.91-2.88)

OR indicates odds ratio; CI, confidence interval; ADL, activities of daily living; and MMSE, Mini-Mental State Examination.

1. Katz S., Ford A.B., et al.: Studies of illness in the aged. The index of ADL: a standardized measure of biological and psychosocial function. *J Am Med Assoc.* 1963;185:914–919.
2. Folstein M.F., Folstein S.E., et al.: "Mini-Mental State": a practical method for grading the cognitive state of patients for the clinician. *J Psychiatr Res.* 1975;12:189–198.
3. Fugl-Meyer AR, Jääskö L, Leyman I, Olsson S, Steglind S. The post-stroke hemiplegic patient, I: a method for evaluation of physical performance. *Scand J Rehabil Med.* 1975;7:13–31.

(continued)

EXAMPLE 3-1 (continued)

Regarding medical disorders, comorbidity conditions, blood component findings, or type or location of brain lesions, no other than those indicated in Table 2 appeared to be associated with the fall risk. As can also be seen, the variables age, previous stroke, previous falls, and orthostatic hypotension did not seem to contribute to the fall risk.

Table 3. Fall Risk Score for Patients in Stroke Rehabilitation

Factor	Score
Sex	
Female	0
Male	2
Katz ADL score[1]	
A-D	0
E-G	2
Urinary continence, Katz ADL categorization[1]	
Independent	0
Dependent (incontinent)	2
Postural stability score[2]	
>=10/14	0
<10/14	1
Signs of motor impairment	
None or unilateral	0
Bilateral	1
Signs of visuospatial hemineglect	
No	0
Yes	1
Bilateral brain lesions including leukoaraiosis	
No	0
Yes	1
Use of diuretics, antidepressants, or sedatives	
No	0
Yes	1

ADL indicates activities of daily living. Scores of factors present are added together to produce an index sum with a maximum of 11.

1. Katz S., Ford A.B., et al.: Studies of illness in the aged. The index of ADL: a standardized measure of biological and psychosocial function. *J Am Med Assoc.* 1963;185:914–919.
2. Fugl-Meyer AR, Jääskö L, Leyman I, Olsson S, Steglind S. The post-stroke hemiplegic patient, I: a method for evaluation of physical performance. *Scand J Rehabil Med.* 1975;7:13–31.

The stepwise Cox regression modeling resulted in the fall risk score presented in Table 3. The weights of the scores were derived from the odds ratios of the final model. As shown, the final model risk factors included male sex, urinary incontinence, Katz ADL score of E or lower, severe postural impairment, bilateral signs of hemiplegia, signs of visuospatial hemineglect, CT-verified bilateral cortical and white matter lesions, and use of diuretics, antidepressants, or sedatives. The variables—high white blood cell count and high blood glucose level—did not contribute significantly to the overall accuracy of the model, nor did the variables dyspraxia or cognitive impairment.

In the total sample, the median fall risk index score was 7, with an interquartile range of 4 to 9 and a total range of 0 to 11. The index score proved to relate significantly to the fall risk in a Cox regression (odds ratio, 1.46; 95% confidence interval, 1.26 to 1.69; Wald 2, 25.13; $P < .001$). The odds ratio indicates that a change of 1 point in the index score related to a 46% increase in the fall risk.

On the basis of distribution of index scores among fallers and nonfallers (Table 4), we suggest the following risk level classifications of the scores: A score from 0 to 4 would indicate a low fall risk, a score of 5 to 7 an

(continued)

EXAMPLE 3-1 (continued)

Table 4. Fall Risk Index Scores Among Patients With and Without Falls During Stroke Rehabilitation

Index Score	Nonfallers (n=86)	Fallers (n=49)
0	4	0
1	4	0
2	6	0
3	13	0
4	11	0
5	9	5
6	9	1
7	10	5
8	6	10
9	9	10
10	3	14
11	2	4

A score of 0–4 would indicate a low fall risk, 5–7 an intermediate risk, and 8–11 a high risk.

intermediate fall risk, and a score of 8 to 11 a high fall risk. The fall risk differed significantly among the patients assigned to the low-, intermediate-, and high-risk groups. No falls occurred among the patients assigned to the low-risk group.

An accurate and easily administered instrument for identifying fall-prone individuals may serve as an important basis for tailored fall reduction models in which reduction measures are directed toward high-risk individuals addressing identified risk factors, either by modification or compensation. Such a reduction approach was recently successfully tested in a community population of elderly persons.

The fall risk index proposed in this study correlated well with the fall risk in a sample of patients in geriatric stroke rehabilitation. Furthermore, we believe that the index suggested offers quite good content validity. The item selection seems suitable for use in a stroke-patient population and reflects established fall risk factors.

The functional items (low ADL score, severe postural stability impairment, and bilateral motor impairment) reflect dependence and reduced locomotion ability and safety. Multifocal or widespread brain lesions can generally be expected to affect neuropsychological function, behavior, and motor abilities. Perceptual impairment is a very likely and often-suggested fall risk factor because it is connected both with attention deficits and impulsivity. Urinary incontinence has previously proved to correlate with rehabilitation outcome, and this factor is assumed to be a marker of the severity of cerebral injury or to reflect a generally low cerebral function level. The reason why the male turned out to be a risk indicator is not clear. There are a few studies indicating that among the institutionalized elderly, men are more likely to fall than women, which is quite contrary to what has uniformly been found in community populations of the elderly. Whether this should be attributed to a supposedly higher degree of proneness to risky behavior or a relatively more pronounced disability among men than women in hospitalized and disabled populations, or some other factors, remains to be determined.

It is noteworthy, however, that the medication factor accounted for an unexpectedly small contribution to the index. Also, cognitive impairment and dyspraxia did not seem to add to the

(continued)

EXAMPLE 3-1 (continued)

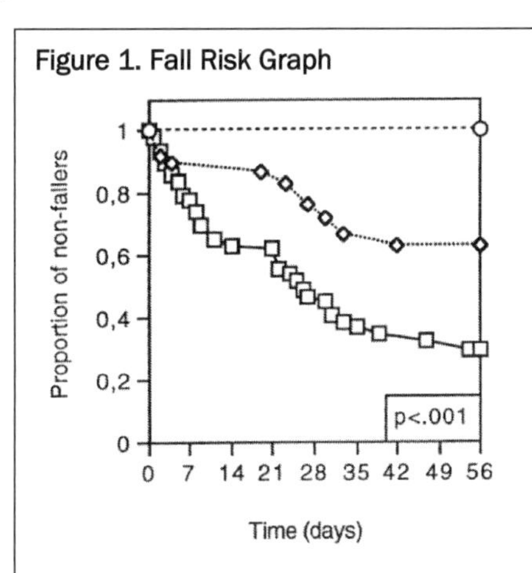

Figure 1. Line graph shows Kaplan-Meier curves for fall risk as a function of time in 135 patients assigned to low-risk (circles and broken line; n = 38), intermediate-risk (diamonds and dotted line; n = 39), and high-risk (squares and solid line; n = 58) groups.

contribution of the other items of the multifactorial model, although these factors were associated with the fall risk in the univariate analyses. Previous (prestroke) falls are likely to be of less importance as a risk indicator in a stroke-patient population because the stroke itself changes the individual's state so dramatically.

Some methodological difficulties were considered in the study design and analyses. Because stroke patients are subject to a considerable amount of change during their acute and subacute phases, the validity of many patient characteristic ratings must be seen as time dependent. Therefore, we limited the study period to a maximum of eight weeks. The fact that the study concerned only the inpatient rehabilitation period resulted in a wide variation in observation time, which was accounted for by the use of survival analysis methods.

The study also had a number of limitations that should be considered. Although completely immobile patients were excluded from the analysis, no specific measure of patient activity was used. Such a measure of the actual risk exposure would undoubtedly have enhanced our analyses. Nor were any measures of increased response time, impulsive behavior, or rightward orienting bias included (for example, factors previously associated with the risk of falls among stroke patients). If these factors had been included, it is possible that our study would have resulted in a better prediction model. The Line-Bisection Test could not be completed by all patients, so some of the ratings regarding visuospatial hemineglect were based on behavioral observations, that were made by an experienced multidisciplinary team constellation. The study included a selected sample of stroke patients. However, we believe that this sample is fairly representative of moderately to severely disabled stroke patients who need further hospital stays and rehabilitation after the acute phase. Furthermore, the accuracy of the fall risk index was expressed only by means of its fit to the data from which it originated. To ensure its accuracy, the index should be tested prospectively on an independent patient sample.

We expect that our proposed index will be easy to administer in the clinical situation. The Katz ADL Index is well known and easily rated by means of information that should be available in the rehabilitation setting. The postural stability score of the Brunnström–Fugl-Meyer assessment includes five well-defined items (two of which are rated bilaterally) and is accomplished in 5 to 10 minutes. Although we assessed bilateral motor impairment using the

(continued)

EXAMPLE 3-1 (continued)

Brunnström–Fugl-Meyer motor score, which is quite elaborate, this could easily be defined as bilateral findings of marked motor impairment (for example, findings indicating more severe impairment than a slight dyscoordination in finger-nose and heel-knee tests or slightly abnormal tendon reflexes). The ratings of visuospatial hemineglect should preferably be accompanied by relevant available testing procedures (for example, the Line Bisection Test). For the time being, we assume that CT scans or other brain imaging techniques are a standard clinical routine in the management of patients with stroke. We therefore expect that the assessment of an index score would not lengthen a standard clinical evaluation by more than approximately 15 to 20 minutes.

This study resulted in a fall prediction model in the form of an index score that correlated very well with the fall risk in a geriatric stroke rehabilitation patient sample. The index is easily administered and intended to be used for patients in stroke rehabilitation. However, its predictive accuracy has to be further evaluated.

Source: American Heart Association, Inc. From the Department of Geriatric Medicine, Umeå University (Sweden).

tends to vary in intensity. For example, examining low-risk senior populations as part of a routine primary health care visit would involve a brief and fairly simple assessment. However, assessing persons with recurrent falls, those living in a nursing home, persons prone to injurious falls, or persons presenting after a fall would call for a more comprehensive and detailed assessment.

In any fall-related assessment, the process must include details about the circumstances of the fall (including a witness account), identification of the subject's risk factors for falls, any medical comorbidity, functional status, and environmental risks.

How do you know that an assessment tool is working well? Continue to collect fall data and analyze it for changes in the fall rate, then ask questions. Piper suggests asking, "Was this person properly identified on the assessment tool? If not, why not? Does something need to be added? Or are staff not actually asking all the questions?" Reassessment of care recipients' physical and psychological status can identify factors that place them at risk for falls. Vigilance in timely assessment is critical in all care settings and with all populations.

In any setting, a health care organization must be prepared to measure the benefits of assessment and intervention—set against the work load and cost implications of a potential increase in referral for specialist assessment—when implementing an assessment plan. The same can be said of the elements, strategies, and mechanisms that support the fall risk assessment process. The chapter ahead considers these issues and others in analyzing the essential aspects of an effective fall reduction program.

References

1. Gaebler S.: Predicting which patients will fall again. *J Adv Nurs* 18:1895–902, 1993.
2. DiBella M., Harvey C.A.: *Falls Decision Tree for Treatment and Prevention.* Washington, DC: Department of Veterans Affairs Virtual Learning Center, 1998.
3. Morse, J.M.: Enhancing the safety of hospitalization by reducing patient falls. *Am J Infect Control* 30:376–380, 2002.
4. Henkel G.: Beyond the MDS: Team approach to falls assessment, prevention, & management. *Caring for the Ages* 3:15–20, Apr. 2002.
5. Joint Commission Resources: Using tools to assess and prevent inpatient falls. *Jt Comm J Qual Safe* 29:365–366, Jul. 2003.
6. Forrester, D.A., et al.: Fall risk assessment of hospitalized adults and follow-up study. *J Nurses Staff Dev* 15:251–258, discussion 258–259, 1999.
7. AGS Panel on Falls Prevention. *JAGS* 49, May 2001.
8. Mayo N.E., et al.: Predicting falls among patients in a rehabilitation hospital. *Am J Phys Med Rehabil* 68:139–146, 1989.
9. Vlahov D., Myers A.H., Al-Ibrahim M.S.: Epidemiology of falls among patients in a rehabilitation hospital. *Arch Phys Med Rehabil* 71:8–12, 1990.
10. Salgado R., et al.: Factors associated with falling in elderly hospital patients. *Gerontology* 40:325–331, 1994.
11. Dromerick A., Reding M.: Medical and neurological complications during inpatient stroke rehabilitation. *Stroke* 25:358–361, 1994.
12. Nyberg L., Gustafson Y. Patient falls in stroke rehabilitation: A challenge to rehabilitation strategies. *Stroke* 26:838–842, 1995.
13. Vellas B., et al.: Prospective study of restriction of activity in old people after falls. *Age Ageing* 16:189–193, 1987.
14. Stein J., Viramontes B.E., Kerrigan D.C.: Fall-related injuries in anticoagulated stroke patients during inpatient rehabilitation. *Arch Phys Med Rehabil* 76:840–843, 1995.
15. Tutuarimia J.A., et al.: Risk factors for falls of hospitalized stroke patients. *Stroke* 28:297–301, 1997.
16. Webster J.S., et al.: Rightward orienting bias, wheelchair maneuvering, and fall risk. *Arch Phys Med Rehabil* 76:924–928, 1995.
17. Forster A., Young J.: Incidence and consequences of falls due to stroke: A systematic inquiry. *BMJ* 311:83–86, 1995.
18. Nevitt M.C., et al.: Risk factors for recurrent nonsyncopal falls: A prospective study. *JAMA* 261:2663–2668, 1989.
19. Tinetti M.E., Speechly M., Ginter S.F.: Risk factors for falls among elderly persons living in the community. *N Engl J Med* 319:1701–1707, 1988.
20. Nyberg L., Gustafson Y.: Using the Downton Index to predict those prone to falls in stroke rehabilitation. *Stroke* 27:1821–1824, 1996.
21. Vellas B.J., et al.: Fear of falling and restriction of mobility in elderly fallers. *Age Ageing* 26:189–193, 1997.
22. Mendes de Leon C.F., et al.: Self-efficacy, physical decline, and change in functioning in community-living elders: A prospective study. *J Gerontol Soc Sci* 51:S183–S190, 1996.
23. Friedman S.M., et al.: Falls and fear of falling: Which comes first? A longitudinal prediction model suggests strategies for primary and secondary prevention. *JAGS* 50:1329–1335, 2002.
24. Downton J.H.: *Falls in the Elderly.* London, UK: Edward Arnold, 1993, pp. 128–130.
25. Gustafson Y.,et al.: Acute confusional states (delirium) in stroke patients. *Cerebrovasc Dis* 1:257–264, 1991.
26. Katz S., et al.: Studies of illness in the aged. The index of ADL: A standardized measure of biological and psychosocial function. *J Am Med Assoc* 185:914–919, 1963.
27. Rubenstein L.Z., Power C.: *Falls and Mobility Problems: Potential Quality Indicators and Literature Review* (the ACOVE Project). Santa Monica, CA: RAND Corp., 1999.
28. Perell K.L.: Assessing the risk of falls: Guidelines for selecting appropriate measures for clinical practice settings. *Generations* pp. 56–68, Winter 2002–2003.
29. Rubenstein L.Z., Josephson K.R., Osterweil D.: Falls and fall prevention in the nursing home. *Clin Geriatr Med* 12:881–903, 1996.
30. King M.B., Tinetti M.E.: A multifactorial approach to reducing injurious falls. *Clin Geriatr Med* 12:745–759, 1996.

31. Tinetti M.E., Williams T.F., Mayewski R.: Fall risk index for elderly patients based on number of chronic disabilities. *Am J Med* 80:429–434, 1986.
32. Wolf-Klein G.P., et al.: Prevention of falls in the elderly population. *Archives of Physical Medicine and Rehabilitation* 69:689–691, 1998.
33. Oliver D., et al.: Development and evaluation of evidence based risk assessment tool (STRATIFY) to predict which elderly inpatients will fall: Case-control and cohort studies. *BMJ* 315:1049–1053, 1997.
34. Hendrich A., et al.: Hospital falls: Development of predictive model for clinical practice. *Appl Nurs Res* 8:129–139, 1995.
35. Rawsky E.: Review of the literature on falls among the elderly. *J Nurs Scholarsh* 30:47–52, 1998.
36. Whitney S.L., Hudak M.T., Marchetti G.F.: The dynamic gait index relates to self-reported fall history in individuals with vestibular dysfunction. *J Vestib Res* 10:199–205, Feb. 2000.
37. Shumway-Cook A., Brauer S., Woollacott M.H.: Predicting the probability for falls in community-dwelling older adults using the timed get up & go test. *Physical Therapy* 80(9): 896–903, 2000.
38. Province M.A., et al.: The effects of exercise on falls and elderly patients: A preplanned meta-analysis of the FICSIT trials. *JAMA* 273: 1341–1347, 1995.
39. Perell K.L., et al.: Fall risk assessment measures: An analytic review. *J Gerontol A Biol Sci Med Sci* 56A:M761–M766, 2001.
40. Morse J. M., Morse. R., Tylko S.: Development of a scale to identify the fall prone patient. *Can J Aging* 8:366–377, 1989.
41. Morse J.M.: *Preventing Patient Falls.* Thousand Oaks, CA: Sage Publications, 1997.
42. Nyberg L., Gustafson Y.: Fall prediction index for patients in stroke rehabilitation. *Stroke* 28:716–721, 1997.

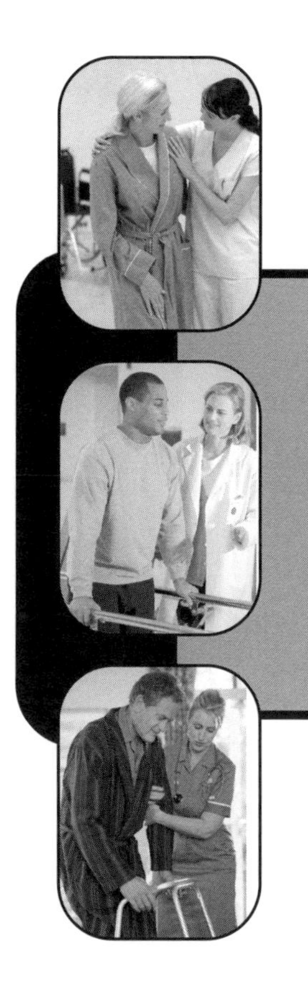

CHAPTER 4

Establishing a Fall Reduction Program

Mrs. Brown is an 89-year-old resident of a skilled nursing facility who uses a walker. She falls in a hallway on her way to the dining room. The floor nurse and a nursing assistant first check her lower extremities for the possibility of a hip fracture. When they determine there is no fracture, they help Mrs. Brown to a nearby bench. Using a short-form checklist, they begin assessing Mrs. Brown for any additional consequences of her fall. They take her blood pressure and pulse and check for swelling, bruising, and pain, as well as change in cognition. They note their findings on the form.

Mrs. Brown states that she is not dizzy and blood pressure readings indicate that she is not hypotensive. She also does not have a history of falling. Moving to other items on the checklist, the nurse and nursing assistant check the immediate environment, noting that the lighting is fine and that there are no spills or obstacles on the floor.

Finally, the nurse checks Mrs. Brown's walker and discovers that one leg is missing its rubber tip. With no other apparent causes pinpointed for the fall, they determine that the damaged walker tip may have been the contributing factor. The walker is sent to maintenance for repair, and Mrs. Brown is given a replacement walker. Staff notify her physician of the fall that day, and after a comprehensive postfall evaluation, Mrs. Brown's care plan is updated to reflect her fall, and her chart is tagged to include more frequent fall risk assessments. In addition, all the walkers in the facility are put on a regular schedule to be checked for repairs.

In this fall incident, did staff follow appropriate procedures in examining the care recipient for injury and assessing the cause of her fall? Did staff properly document their findings? Did staff communicate their findings appropriately? Did staff adjust the care recipient's fall status? Did staff apply their findings to the entire facility?

In this case, the answers are "yes." Each question posed offers an inquiry into the elements of an effective fall reduction program, and the example above provides evidence of staff initiating a systematic procedure to properly address a care recipient fall. In this scenario, steps that include checklists, examination, documentation, and communication all converge into a plan of action.

As the previous chapter outlined, the beginning stages in building a comprehensive fall reduction program include assembling an interdisciplinary team and applying risk assessment tools that will help determine effective intervention strategies. In widening the scope on the issue of care recipient falls, this chapter begins with a review of the fundamental aspects of an effective fall reduction program before more thoroughly analyzing the principles and procedures of the intervention process. Including specific interventions for care recipients at risk of falling, the use of data in developing intervention strategies, the ways in which research and decision making apply to intervention planning, and the importance of institutional support for intervention strategies, this chapter examines the elements that drive the overarching goal of any fall reduction program: to reduce care recipient falls and minimize the risk of injury when a fall occurs.

The Principles of a Fall Reduction Program

Studies have shown that both falls and injuries can be reduced through an effective program. For health care organizations, the process of addressing fall reduction is similar to that of other clinical problems. That process should include the following three primary steps:

1. Identify and evaluate all care recipient fall occurrences.
2. Establish a process for fall reduction.
3. Monitor the program's effectiveness, including staff compliance.[1]

Identify Fall Occurrences

Before a program can be developed, it is important that an organization collect and analyze data to determine when, where, and why falls are occurring. Incident reports can provide a comprehensive picture of fall occurrences both in care recipient homes and on inpatient units.

The data collected from incident reports will provide information on the following:

- Number of falls (for example, overall and at specific times of day and day of week)
- Type of fall (for example, while ambulating, from bed, from chair, found on floor, during transfer)
- Location of fall (for example, room, bathroom, hall)
- Care recipient mental status at time of fall (for example, oriented, confused, medicated)
- Safety measures in use at time of fall (for example, bed in low position, wheelchair seat belt secured [if applicable], call bell within reach, bed or chair alarm on)
- Injury sustained, type and severity

Performing a risk analysis of falls can help identify trends that could contribute to the frequency of falls and direct staff toward potential measures to reduce falls. Because every organization is different, fall data are best used as an internal barometer of a program's success rather than as a measurement of comparison with another organization.

Home care fall incidents are more difficult to evaluate than those in a facility because falls often occur when agency staff are not on site.

Home care recipients may not report such falls, especially if there is no injury. To better evaluate at-home falls, care recipients should be encouraged to report all falls, even when there is no injury.

Although statistics provide an overview of fall occurrences, they do not provide a complete picture of a specific fall. Performing an investigation can identify contributing factors such as understaffing, failure to follow procedures, and the existence of an unsafe condition, as well as ways to reduce future occurrences.

The American Medical Directors Association's (AMDA) Falls and Fall Risk Clinical Practice Guideline (CPG) urges facility administrators to incorporate analysis of falls into quality-improvement studies. Tracking falls on a monthly basis can allow the medical director to pinpoint environmental causes of falls.

For instance, at one facility a medical director noticed a rise in falls in July and August on certain units. After performing a root cause analysis, the medical director and the facility's administrators determined that nurses were taking more vacations in July and August. Temporary nurses had not been trained adequately in fall reduction. The solution was to stagger nurses' vacations so that more experienced nurses were always available to inform replacement staff of the procedures.[2]

Establish a Process to Reduce Falls

A systematic and organized approach to fall reduction can help in focusing resources on those who are at the greatest risk for a fall. In establishing, following, and documenting fall reduction procedures, an organization can demonstrate that it has taken reasonable measures to protect its care recipients from harm. Such procedures can even be used as a defense to mitigate liability damages in a claim involving alleged damages from a fall incident.

As outlined in Chapter 3, the use of risk assessment data is an effective way to identify care recipients who are at a high risk. All care recipients should be assessed for fall risk upon admission, with reassessments performed as indicated by established criteria for the following occurrences:

- Fall incident
- Change in medical condition
- Change in mental status
- Change in mobility

In addition to performing a fall assessment upon admission, the home environment should be evaluated for safety exposures that could contribute to a fall.

Care Recipient Safety Measures

Part of establishing a consistent approach to reducing falls involves instituting care recipient safety measures that appropriate staff members initiate whenever a care recipient has been identified as a fall risk. Safety guidelines employed to reduce fall frequency can include the following:

- Identify care recipients who are at high risk of a fall and alert staff to these care recipients. Some systems employ a special identification system that includes marking the rooms of high-risk care recipients. Fall risk status should always be visibly identified on the care recipient's chart.
- Educate the care recipient and his or her family to the risk and to the need to always call for assistance before attempting to get up.
- Monitor care recipient needs on a regular basis (at least every two hours).
- Place the bed in the lowest position when not providing care.
- Make sure the call bell is always within the

care recipient's reach while in bed, in a chair, or in the bathroom.

- Anticipate care recipient needs; keep water, tissue, urinal, and so forth within easy reach.
- Keep the top bed rail up (beds with quarter rails) to assist the care recipient in getting to a sitting position.
- Use bed and chair pressure-sensitive alarms for care recipients who do not follow directions or refuse to request assistance.
- Use seat belts in wheelchairs.
- Use side rails when transporting a care recipient on a cart as applicable.
- Always use wheelchair brakes and bed wheel locks when performing a transfer.

All efforts to identify and protect at-risk care recipients should be documented in the medical record. A well-documented medical record will do the following:

- Provide for clear communication between all caregivers.
- Permit more comprehensive performance improvement reviews.
- Offer evidence that reasonable care was taken to protect a care recipient from injury when there is a claim as the result of a fall incident.

In the AMDA's CPG report, which provides an outline for facilities developing their own fall reduction programs, health care organizations have room to customize their own processes to fit their facility. The AMDA's guidelines include the following process indicators for development of fall reduction programs:

- Fall risk assessment should be documented for each new admission.
- A physician should address any medical or medication risk factors in someone identified as being at moderate or high risk of falling.
- A physician should review the case of any care recipient who falls more than once or who has a fall with a significant injury for potentially correctable conditions or problems.
- Evaluation of factors (environment, staffing, time of day) associated with actual falls should be done.
- A physician should modify any medications or treatments that are commonly associated with falling or explain why doing so is not indicated.

Educate and Train Staff

As discussed in the previous chapter, staff training is key to an effective fall reduction program. Training should focus on following program procedures, maintaining a safe environment, and using proper lifting and transferring techniques.

Program Monitoring

No program is complete unless it includes a component to perform ongoing monitoring of its effectiveness. As in the initial fall risk analysis, data collected through incident and occurrence reporting provide a basis for this oversight, offering a better understanding of why falls are taking place and what strategies might counteract them.

It is not possible to prevent falls, nor is it possible to arrive at a root cause for every fall. However, a well-designed, well-documented, and consistently followed reduction process can achieve its most important goal: to reduce the risk of falls and minimize the risk of injury when a fall occurs.

The Principles of Intervention

As discussed in Chapter 3, researcher Janice Morse categorizes falls as accidental, unanticipated physiologic, or anticipated physiologic.

SIDEBAR 4-1

Result-Oriented Interventions

Medicine
- Risk assessment and identification (for example, joint and balance testing, muscle strength testing)
- Medication evaluation
- Medical intervention for acute and chronic conditions

Nursing
- Risk-factor screening
- Care planning for risk factors
- Transfer and gait training
- Muscle-strengthening exercises
- Provide ambulation aids.
- Provide proper footwear.
- Provide pressure-graded stockings.
- Investigate falls and suggest precautionary measures.
- Maintain proper staffing.
- Maintain proper supervision (particularly at peak activity/accident time and shift changes).

Occupational Therapy
- Provide chairs with arms, proper height.
- Provide toilet pillows to raise seats.
- Provide cervical collars.

Therapeutic Recreation
- Exercise classes
- Motivation therapy
- Sensory stimulation

Social Services
- Provide psychosocial intervention with residents and families.

Optometry/Ophthalmology
- Vision screening
- Provide glasses/lenses.
- Eye care, cataract extraction

Audiology/ENT
- Audiological screening
- Provide hearing aids.

Podiatry
- Foot and nail care

Administration
- Provide facility philosophy, policy, and direction.

Maintenance
- Paint edges of stairs in bright colors to help with depth-perception problems.
- Install and maintain handrails at proper height.
- Install adequate glare-free day-and-night lighting.
- Use nonglare paint on walls.
- Highlight night switches.
- Install and maintain grab bars on toilets and tubs.
- Install high toilet seats.

Housekeeping
- Maintain dry nonskid, nonshiny floors.
- Position furniture in nonobstructing patterns.
- Avoid placing obstacles while cleaning.
- Provide proper clothing.

Physical or Occupational Therapy
- Provide proper shoes.
- Provide and monitor ambulation devices.
- Provide advice on procurement of all seating equipment.
- Provide and monitor all seating equipment.

In-Service
- Provide transfer and ambulation training to reduce the risk of an accident that may occur during transfer.
- Assure staff that no disciplinary action will be taken if an accident occurs while policies and procedures are properly followed.
- Encourage staff to report accidents in a timely manner to assure proper care.

Medical Director/Nursing Director
- Monitor all accidents to identify possible hazards and formulate corrective action.[3]

Morse also contends that fall interventions must be linked to each etiologic factor.[4]

Accidental falls can be reduced by ensuring a safe environment. For example, following a checklist that includes fitting care recipients with nonskid footwear, ensuring that spills are immediately wiped up, routinely checking and repairing equipment, and making sure handrails are appropriately placed are among the measures that can help reduce care recipient falls.

Because the first unanticipated physiologic fall is, by definition, unexpected, it cannot be prevented. Depending on the cause, subsequent falls may not be prevented. In this event, the goal is to protect the care recipient from injury should a fall recur. According to Morse, protective strategies are individualized and include such measures as teaching the care recipient how to fall safely and how to rise from a prone position slowly, and by providing helmets.

Interventions for care recipients considered at risk of an anticipated physiologic fall are both protective and precautionary. The protective strategies that must be provided immediately include the following:

- Increased observation to provide appropriate assistance with ambulation
- Bed alarms (which are intended to alert staff to provide assistance before the care recipient gets out of bed)
- Establishment of routines such as regular toileting (so that the care recipient will not become restless and try to get out of bed alone)
- Teaching of protective behaviors (for example, teaching a care recipient how to fall or to transfer safely)
- Devices to assist with ambulation (for example, walkers and handrails)
- Devices to minimize injury if the care recipient does fall (for example, hip protectors and helmets)

Precautionary strategies are also used with care recipients who are at risk for anticipated physiologic falls. These strategies are designed to reduce fall risk. This goal is most often accomplished through the use of a more detailed fall assessment that can identify specific interventions. For example, for a care recipient who requires a gait assessment, the interventions identified may include physical therapy or a new type of walking aid to help improve mobility.

The Differences Between Protection and Intervention

Morse also points out the importance of distinguishing between fall protection and fall intervention.

Protective strategies are primarily the responsibility of nurses, according to Morse. These strategies are intended to reduce an imminent fall or, if the care recipient does fall, to protect the care recipient from injury. It follows, then, that the care recipient should be assessed to identify appropriate protective strategies on admission and reassessed upon any change of condition. Or, if a fall does occur, the care recipient should be assessed and reassessed to help determine a care plan to protect the care recipient from a second fall. This is particularly important because repeated falls are not uncommon. Morse found that 69% of care recipients who experienced more than one fall in a rehabilitation hospital were engaging in the same activity during the next fall.

Protective strategies must be immediate and responsive to care recipient needs because the availability of adequate protective strategies will make the greatest difference in reducing fall and injury rates. Protective strategies also require resources such as adequate staffing, and health care organizations must budget accordingly for the costs of fall interventions. Care recipients who refuse to use their call bell and continue to climb out of bed despite warnings may be protected from injury if a staff member remains with the care recipient or if a bed alarm is placed on the bed. Another example that requires adequate staffing is the waking of care recipients for toileting at regular intervals during the night.

Fall-protective care plans must be individualized and evidence based. The policies of health care organizations should dictate personalized assessment because strategies intended to protect one care recipient may place another at risk. For example, if side rails are used to remind the care recipient where the edge of the bed is, they are used to protect the care recipient from rolling out of bed. However, if the side rails are intended to keep a restless care recipient in bed, they may increase the risk of injury because the care recipient may attempt to climb over the side rail or the end of the bed, or may try to force himself or herself through the rails. Evidence, not custom or habit, should determine the appropriate interventions for a care recipient. Otherwise, side rails that are intended to reduce falls, for example, may instead decrease mobility, increase the risk of falling and injury, and contribute to mortality.

Intervention strategies, on the other hand, do not usually have an immediate effect (as in the case of reducing the fall risk of an anticipated physiologic fall) or are not targeted directly to a specific care recipient (as in the case of an accidental fall). Fall assessments are designed to determine physiologic problems that may result in a fall—primarily those that interfere with gait or mental status. Some assessments require special equipment, such as an isokinetic dynamometer to evaluate muscle strength, or specific measurement tools, such as the Activities of Daily Vision Scale.

Fall assessments do not substitute for predictive scales that determine the risk of falling. One group of researchers concluded that efforts to predict falls are less beneficial than a program of education and fall reduction when an assessment tool is mistakenly used rather than a predictive risk scale. However, because the majority of falls can be anticipated and linked to particular risk factors, it is essential to use reliable and valid instruments for fall risk in order to implement corresponding interventions.

Interventions for All Care Recipients

Although the outcome analyses of a risk assessment process help determine intervention strategies specific to individual care recipients, there are many interventions an organization can adopt to reduce the likelihood of falls for all care recipients.

Reviewing Environmental Risk Factors

In previous chapters, and as noted by Morse above, the effort of reducing care recipient falls relies in great part on the vigilance of staff to ensure a safe environment of care. Even the way in which furniture and equipment is arranged in a care recipient's room can make an impact on reducing the risk of falls. Although the setup of a care recipient's room can be individualized for that care recipient, there are some general setup principles for all care recipients, regardless of risk.

As outlined in the National Center for Patient Safety (NCPS) Toolkit, each care recipient should be assigned to a bed that allows exit toward his or her stronger side, and the care recipient's bedside table, call bell, and light switch should be within his or her reach. All rooms should be well lit and free of clutter and tripping hazards. All bathroom and exit doors should be clearly marked with both letters and pictures. All movable equipment should be locked. The furniture should be both sturdy and comfortable, and beds should be adjustable in height.[5]

Care recipients determined to be at high risk for falls should be assigned to rooms as close to the nurses' station as possible. Nonslip padded flooring or floor mats should be placed on the exit side of the bed. Devices that mark bed boundaries, such as concave mattresses, should be considered. Handrails should be accessible and sturdy, and walking aids, transfer bars, bedside commodes, and other assistive devices should be located on the exit side of the bed.

Because many falls occur in the bathroom and shower areas, many organizations focus more aggressively on details in the bathroom. For example, they use slip-resistant strips in the tub and on the bathroom floor as well as a cleanser that increases traction even when wet, install toilet transfer bars at a height appropriate for the care recipient, and place a stool in the shower for care recipients to sit on.

An organization should set in place interventions to ensure that both care recipients and staff can move freely and safely in hallways. Hallways should remain free of clutter, unused equipment, or tripping hazards such as electrical cords. They should always be well lit, and broken lights should be fixed promptly. Handrails in hallways should be accessible and sturdy, and, when possible, chairs should be set in hallways as periodic rest stops.

Some organizations have chosen to place two high-risk care recipients in a two-bed room so that they can watch each other when moving around. Other rooms accommodating high-risk care recipients have a window so staff can keep watch over care recipients without disturbing them.

Another important way to reduce hazards in the environment is to be thorough in conducting environmental and equipment assessments. They should be done frequently and encompass a wide variety of areas, from securing door handles and ensuring that the flooring is level between door thresholds, to ensuring that bed adjustments work properly and rubber tips are securely fastened to the bottom of canes and walkers.

To aid staff in conducting environmental assessments, some facilities have developed checklists for staff. The example of Janice Morse's equipment checklist in Figure 4-1 has been modified to include updated technology.[6]

As mentioned previously, even simple procedures such as requiring care recipients to wear treaded slipper socks or shoes when they are up and moving around can lessen the chance of a fall. The exception in this case is if the facility is carpeted throughout. When on carpet, care recipients should not wear treaded slipper socks because this could increase their likelihood of falling, especially if they shuffle their feet while walking.

When care recipients are unfamiliar with their environment, they are more likely to trip and have difficulty moving around. Implementing an easy process that makes them more aware of their surroundings will be beneficial to their activities. Care recipients should also gain an understanding of how to use assistive devices prior to using them and be given proper and thorough instruction about their medications, from times and dosages to side effects and interactions with food and other medications.

As outlined in Chapter 1, Goal 8 of the Joint Commission's National Patient Safety Goals focuses on the importance of documenting medications across the continuum of care. Sidebar 4-2 on page 90 offers compliance suggestions that relate to this goal.

Even if a care recipient is not considered at high risk for a fall, his or her condition can change, increasing the likelihood of falling. Staff should monitor a care recipient's risk fac-

FIGURE 4-1

Equipment Safety Confirmation

Equipment Safety Checklist

Item	Check	
Wheelchairs		
Brakes	Secure chair when applied	______
Arm rest	Detaches easily for transfers	______
Leg rest	Adjusts easily	______
Foot pedals	Fold easily so that patient may stand	______
Wheels	Are not bent or warped	______
Antitip devices	Installed, placed in proper position	______
Electric Wheelchairs/Scooters		
Speed	Set at lowest setting	______
Horn	Works properly	______
Electrical	Wires are not exposed	______
Beds		
Side rails	Raise and lower easily	______
	Secure when up	______
Wheels	Roll/turn easily, do not stick	______
Brakes	Secure the bed firmly when applied	______
Mechanics	Height adjusts easily (if applicable)	______
Transfer bars	Sturdy, attached properly	______
Over-bed table	Wheels firmly locked	______
	Positioned on wall-side of bed	______
IV Poles/Stands		
Pole	Raises/lowers easily	______
Wheels	Roll easily and turn freely, do not stick	______
Stand	Stable, does not tip easily (should be five-point base)	______
Footstools		
Legs	Rubber skid protectors on all feet	______
	Steady—does not rock	______
Top	Nonskid surface	______
Call Bells/Lights		
Operational	Outside door light	______
	Sounds at nursing station	______
	Room number appears on the monitor	______
	Intercom	______
	Room panel signals	______
Accessible	Accessible in bathroom	______
	Within reach while patient is in bed	______
Walkers/Canes		
Secure	Rubber tips in good condition?	______
	Unit is stable	______
Commode		
Wheels	Roll/turn easily, do not stick	______
	Are weighted and not "top heavy" when a patient is sitting on it	______
Brakes	Secure commode when applied	______
Geri/Broda Chairs		
Chair	Located on level surface to minimize risk of tipping	______
Wheels	Roll/turn easily, do not stick	______
Brakes	Applied when chair is stationary	______
	Secure chair firmly when applied	______
Footplate	Removed when chair is placed in a nontilt or nonreclined position	______
	Removed during transfers	______
Positioning	Chair is positioned with proper amount of tilt to prevent sliding or falling forward	______
Tray	Secure	______

SIDEBAR 4-2

Joint Commission National Patient Safety Goal

NEW! *Goal 8: Accurately and completely reconcile medications across the continuum of care.*

Compliance Suggestions

To comply with this goal and its requirements, an organization should develop a standardized method for creating an accurate list of medications at admission and transfer. Development of a medication reconciliation form, to be used as a template for gathering information about current medications, is one method that can be used to standardize care and avoid errors. A specific staff member should be assigned the responsibility of filling out the medication reconciliation form; this person should address all discrepancies and issues with the list. In this way, one person knows everything about a care recipient's medication list, rather than several staff members knowing partial pieces of the care recipient's list. The care recipient's accurate medication reconciliation form (complete with medications prescribed by the first provider of service) is communicated to the next provider of service, whether within or outside the organization. Thereafter, the next provider of service should check over the medication reconciliation form again to make sure it is accurate.

The following tips will also help boost compliance:

- Although obtaining a copy of a medication profile (from the pharmacy or home health agency or other organization that the care recipient was transferred from) is a good initial source of information, verify it with the care recipient and/or the care recipient's family. Sometimes these documents are not up to date or accurate, and the care recipient might have new information.
- If the care recipient was in ambulatory care prior to admission, conduct a "brown bag" review of the care recipient's current medications. Ask the care recipient's family to bring in all the care recipient's home medications so that they can be reviewed.
- When conducting a care recipient interview about medications taken, do not forget over-the-counter drugs, herbals, and dietary supplements. Care recipients may not view these as "medications," but they are.
- Develop an internal and external transfer summary and discharge referral form for the nurse to complete. This form should contain vital information about the care recipient, including a complete list of medications the care recipient is receiving at discharge or transfer. This information should then be sent to the next level of care or the next health care organization.
- Eliminate writing discharge prescriptions on blank prescription pads, a copy of which is not retained in the medical record. Have a form for the physician to complete, which can be used to document the medications ordered on discharge for the medical record, and another form to be used as the prescription for an outside pharmacy to fill.
- It is particularly important in home care (for example, home infusion) for the home health agency to share its assessment information with the dispensing pharmacy, and for the pharmacy to share any medication profile it has on record with the home health agency.

tors frequently, upon transfer, and whenever his or her status changes. According to the NCPS Falls Toolkit, this includes the following:

- Evaluate and treat gait changes, postural instability, and spasticity.
- Evaluate and treat care recipients for impaired vision and hearing.
- Evaluate medications for factors that increase

the risk of falling (for example, use of antihypotensives, psychotropic medications and drug interactions).

- Evaluate and treat pain.
- Evaluate and treat orthostatic hypotension.
- Assess and treat impaired central processing (dementia, delirium, stroke, and perception).

Individual Interventions for High-Risk Care Recipients

For those who are considered to be at high risk for falls, there are other aspects of intervention that can be applied. Before looking at specific measures that relate to an individual, it is important to consider interventions that apply to all high-risk care recipients. Again, in all high-risk cases the room arrangement should follow a predetermined setup, and medications should be reviewed.

For those who have experienced frequent falls, hip protectors that protect hip fractures should be considered. They might also be evaluated further through rehabilitation therapy. For care recipients who experience incontinence, nocturia, or urgency, an individualized toileting schedule can be initiated, and particular medication for reducing urgency might be recommended. For care recipients with dizziness or vertigo, it is important to monitor and treat orthostatic hypotension. Care recipients should also be taught to rise from bed slowly to prevent fainting.

For care recipients experiencing cognitive/memory problems—this includes care recipients who forget their limitations—the NCPS Toolkit recommends the following interventions:

- *Bed and chair alarms.* These alarms can be used to alert the staff when a care recipient is attempting to transfer on his or her own. There are two types of alarms: pressure sensor alarms (when the weight of a care recipient is removed from the sensor, the alarm sounds) and tab alarms (when the care recipient moves beyond the length of the string attached to them, the alarm sounds). Both of these alarms can be hooked up to the nurse call system and can sound at the nursing station.
- *Bed placement.* The bed can be placed along the wall so that the care recipient exits toward their stronger side. This eliminates the need for side rails, reducing the likelihood of bed entrapment.
- *Hip protectors.* Hip protectors are a good intervention for care recipients with dementia and other cognitive defects. They allow the care recipient to be active while helping to prevent hip fractures if they fall. Generally, care recipients should wear them all the time, but some care recipients may find them uncomfortable at night.
- *Frequent checks on the care recipient.* The care recipient should be checked on frequently if in his or her room. If the care recipient is prone to wandering, a safe place should be provided that is supervised and set up with comfortable chairs and handrails.

When care recipients with cognitive impairments use mobility aids, several things should be done to ensure that the care recipient knows how and remembers to use the aid. Mobility aids should be placed directly next to the care recipient's bed on the side that the care recipient exits. Care recipients should use the mobility aid frequently to increase the likelihood that they will remember how to use it. To assess a care recipient's knowledge of how to use a mobility aid, ask him or her to use it—not to explain how to use it. Even if a care recipient cannot explain how to use the mobility aid, he or she may be able to use it.

Indicators and Interventions for Those with Mobility Problems

Impaired gait and balance rank among the most significant underlying causes of falls. They are also common consequences of falls. Because older adults often do not report these problems to physicians, they may go undetected until after injury and disabilities have occurred.

In addition to reducing function and causing considerable morbidity and mortality, falls and instability precipitate premature nursing home admission.[7]

Detectable gait abnormalities affect 20% to 40% of persons 65 years of age or older. Approximately half of those in this group have a grossly abnormal gait. Gait problems are reported to be even more common in older subgroups. In a large study of community-living persons 75 years of age and older, 10% needed assistance to walk across a room, 20% were unable to climb a flight of stairs without help, and 40% were unable to walk a half mile.[8]

"Falls and mobility problems generally result from multiple, diverse, and interacting causes," according to a report by Laurence Z. Rubenstein, M.D., M.P.H., and others, titled "Quality Indicators for the Management and Prevention of Falls and Mobility Problems in Vulnerable Elders." "After detecting a problem, clinicians must use careful and thorough diagnostic approaches to identify the most likely cause, contributing factors, and associated comorbid conditions, many of which will respond to intervention," states the report.

Several clinical approaches have been forwarded as measures to address the complex and serious concerns of falls and mobility problems in older persons. Rubenstein has grouped the approaches that have been demonstrated as effective through quality indicators into three categories: (1) detection of the problem or problems, (2) diagnosis or evaluation of the problem or problems, and (3) treatment, with an aim toward preventing recurrence.

Six indicators of these care processes were judged sufficiently valid for use as measures of the quality of fall and mobility disorder management for vulnerable elders. Rubenstein suggests that these quality indicators (listed below) can potentially serve as a basis with which to compare the care provided by different health care delivery systems and the change in care over time.

Quality Indicator 1—Inquiring about falls. All vulnerable elders should have documentation that they were asked at least annually about the occurrence of recent falls because falls are common, frequently unreported, and often the cause of injury and unnecessary restriction of activity, which results in a reduction in overall health and quality of life. In addition, a recent history of falls is a strong predictor of future falls.

Rubenstein notes, "In addition to causing injury, falls can be strong indicators of accelerating frailty and the presence of underlying, treatable risk factors." He also states that if no injury has occurred, "care recipients and providers alike often ignore falls, thus missing important opportunities for potentially life-saving evaluation and treatment. Inquiring regularly about recent falls can help detect this risk factor and lead to appropriate intervention. One study has shown that fewer falls go undetected (that is, fewer persons who fall are mislabeled as persons who do not fall) when the care recipient is asked about falls that occurred in the previous one-year period than when he or she is asked about a shorter period, such as six months."

Quality Indicator 2—Detecting balance and gait disturbances. All vulnerable elders should have documentation that they were asked about or examined for the presence of balance or gait disturbances at least once because normal balance or gait disturbances are important to health and quality of life, and underlying, treatable problems often go undetected.

Quality Indicator 3—Basic fall evaluation. If a vulnerable elder reports two or more falls in the past year, or a single fall with injury requiring treatment, then there should be documentation that a basic fall evaluation was performed that resulted in specific diagnostic and therapeutic recommendations. Many causes of falls can be detected and treated, and detection and treatment will reduce the likelihood of future falls and associated complications.

Quality Indicator 4—Gait mobility and balance evaluation. If a vulnerable elder reports or is found to have new or worsening difficulty with ambulation, balance, or mobility, then there should be documentation that a basic gait, mobility, and balance evaluation was performed within six months that resulted in specific diagnostic and therapeutic recommendations. Many causes of gait and mobility disturbances can be detected and treated, often by prescribing specific assistive devices and exercises that will reduce the likelihood of future falls and their associated complications.

Rubenstein also notes that several studies have shown that it is important to evaluate mobility problems[9–11]: "A careful examination can detect many contributors to abnormal mobility (for example, muscle weakness, joint abnormalities, neurological dysfunction, pain, postural hypotension), most of which respond favorably to treatment. For example, gait problems related to muscle weakness improve with strengthening exercises, and balance problems improve with specific balance training."

Quality Indicator 5—Exercise and assistive-device prescription for balance problems. If a vulnerable elder demonstrates decreased balance or increased postural sway, then an appropriate exercise program should be offered and an evaluation for an assistive device performed. Impaired balance or proprioception and increased postural sway can contribute to instability, and appropriate treatment will reduce the likelihood of falls and their complications.

Quality Indicator 6—Exercise prescription for gait problems and weakness. If a vulnerable elder is found to have problems with gait, strength (for example ≤4 out of 5 on manual muscle testing, or the need to use his or her arms to rise from a chair), then an exercise program should be offered. These problems can contribute to falls and mobility dysfunction, and exercise intervention can improve or ameliorate them and reduce the likelihood of falls and their complications.

Rubenstein concludes his report by noting, "Falls and mobility problems are generally the result of multiple, diverse, and interacting causes. Falls and gait disorders represent an underlying pathologic condition that may be amenable to treatment but may herald clinical demise if left unrecognized. Improvements in processes of care for falls in this high-risk population may lead to substantial improvements in care recipient outcomes."

Generally, a fear of falling is rooted in some balance or mobility issues. It is recommended that care recipients with a fear of falling have a balance/strength assessment done by a physical or occupational therapist. Additional interventions for those who fear falling can include hip protectors—especially if the care recipient is frail or at high risk of fracture—and lowering the bed to a very low position to reduce the distance the care recipient would fall while getting out of bed.

The NCPS Toolkit lists the following five interventions to consider for care recipients who have gait or mobility problems:

1. Have an occupational therapist (OT)

assess the environment and implement his or her recommendations. Often an OT will recommend aids such as transfer bars or raised toilet seats that are based on the individual needs of the care recipient.

2. Have a physical therapist or occupational therapist assess the care recipient and implement his or her recommendations. It is important that nursing staff comply with the exercise program because exercise programs have been shown to reduce falls as part of a multifaceted fall reduction program.

3. Place a commode next to the bed if the care recipient has difficulty walking to the bathroom at night.

4. Care recipients who are unable to get out of bed or ambulate on their own should have the bed in a very low position to make it harder to get out of bed without assistance.

5. Care recipients should be assisted with toileting as needed.

If an individual assessment for an exercise program is not feasible, staff might institute exercise programs that focus strictly on balance.

Approaches to Care Recipient Lifting and Repositioning

When it comes to procedures that involve care recipient transfers and the National Patient Safety Goal requirement that applicable programs must have a transfer protocol, health care organizations must consider many issues in ensuring care recipient safety and staff safety. According to research from the U.S. Department of Labor's Occupational Safety & Health Administration (OSHA), organizations that implement injury reduction efforts focusing on care recipient lifting and repositioning methods can achieve considerable success in reducing work-related injuries and associated workers' compensation costs. Providing a safer and more comfortable work environment can also result in additional benefits for some facilities, including reduced staff turnover and associated training and administrative costs, reduced absenteeism, increased productivity, improved employee morale, and increased care recipient comfort.[12]

Because care recipient lifting and repositioning tasks can be variable and unpredictable in nature, specific techniques have been developed for assessing these tasks. An analysis of any care recipient lifting and repositioning task involves an assessment of the needs and abilities of the care recipient involved. In this assessment, staff members take into account care recipient characteristics while determining the safest methods for performing the task. This determination, of course, should be within the context of a care plan that provides for appropriate care and services for the care recipient. Such assessments typically consider the safety, dignity, and other rights of the care recipient, as well as the need to maintain or restore functional abilities. The care recipient assessment should include an examination of the following:

- Level of assistance the care recipient requires
- Size and weight of the care recipient
- Ability and willingness of the care recipient to understand and cooperate
- Any medical conditions that may influence the choice of methods for lifting or repositioning

These factors are critical in determining appropriate methods for lifting and repositioning a care recipient. In some cases, the size and weight of the care recipient will determine which equipment is needed and how many caregivers are required to provide assistance. The care recipient's physical and mental abilities are also important to consider in selecting appropriate solutions. For example, a care recipient who is able and willing to partially support his or her own weight may be able to move from the bed to a chair using a standing assist device, while a mechanical sling lift may be more appropriate for those care recipients who are unable to support their own weight. Other conditional factors may need to be taken into account as well. For example, a care recipient who has recently undergone hip replacement surgery may require specialized equipment for assistance in order to avoid placing stress on the affected area.

A number of protocols have been developed for systematically examining care recipient needs and abilities and/or for recommending procedures and equipment to be used for performing lifting and repositioning tasks.

In a nursing home, many individuals can contribute to care recipient assessment and the determination of appropriate methods for assisting in transfer or repositioning. Interdisciplinary teams such as staff nurses, certified nursing assistants, nursing supervisors, physical therapists, physicians, and the care recipient or his/her representative may all be involved. Because the needs and abilities of care recipients may vary considerably over a short period of time, the employees directly responsible for providing assistance are in the best position to be aware of and able to accommodate such changes.

Implementing Solutions for Care Recipient Lifting and Repositioning

Although OSHA has recommended solutions for care recipient lifting and repositioning in the illustrations ahead, it is not expected that all of them will be used in any given facility. They are offered only as a range of available options that a facility can consider using.

According to OSHA, the integration of various solutions into a health care facility is a strategic decision that, if carefully planned and executed, can lead to long-term benefits. Administrators should be cognizant of several factors that might restrict the application of certain measures, such as care recipients' rehabilitation plans, the need for restoration of functional abilities, other medical contraindications, emergency conditions, and the care recipients' dignity and rights.

Administrators should also be aware that the procurement of equipment and the selection of an equipment supplier are important considerations when implementing solutions. Establishing close working relationships with equipment suppliers can help with obtaining training for employees, modifying the equipment for special circumstances, and procuring parts and service when needed. Employers should pay particular attention to the effectiveness of the equipment, especially the injury and illness experience of other facilities that have used the equipment. The following questions can assist in the process of selecting equipment and suppliers that best meet the needs of an individual organization:

- Availability of technical service. Is over-the-phone assistance, as well as on-site assistance, available for repairs and service of the lift?
- Availability of parts. Which parts will be in stock and available in a short time frame, and how soon can they be shipped to your location?
- Storage requirements. Is the equipment too big for your facility? Can it be stored in close proximity to the area(s) where it is used?
- If needed, is a charging unit and backup battery included? Is the charging unit simple to operate? How much space is required for a battery charger if one is needed?
- If the lift has a self-contained charging unit, how much space is necessary for charging,

and what electrical receptacles are required? What is the minimum charging time of a battery?

- How high is the base of the lift, and will it fit under the bed and various other pieces of furniture? How wide is the base of the lift, or is it adjustable to a wider and lockable position?
- How many people are required to operate the lift for lifting a typical 200-lb. person?
- Does the lift activation device (pendant) have remote capabilities?
- How many sizes and types of slings are available? What type of sling is available for optimum infection control?
- Is the device versatile? Can it be a sit-to-stand lift, as well as a lift device? Can it be a sit-to-stand lift and an ambulation-assist device?
- What is the speed and noise level of the device? Will the lift go to floor level? How high will it go?

Considering many factors, including the characteristics of the care recipient population and the layout of the facility, employers should determine the number and types of devices needed. Devices should be located so that they are easily accessible to workers. If care recipient lifting equipment is not accessible when it is needed, it is likely that other aspects of the ergonomics process will be affected. If the facility can initially purchase only a portion of the equipment needed, it should be located in the areas where the needs are greatest. Employers should also establish routine maintenance schedules to ensure that the equipment is in good working order. Figures 4-2, 4-3, 4-4, 4-5, 4-6, and 4-7 are examples of solutions for care recipient lifting and repositioning tasks developed by OSHA.

Consider Caregiver Safety in Care Recipient Transfers

The tasks involved in repositioning a care recipient can take a physical toll on health care staff. Manual lifting and other physical demands are associated with an increased risk of pain and injury to caregivers, particularly to the back.[13] Health care workers involved with care recipient care transfers face risk factors that include the following:

- Force—the amount of physical effort required to perform a task (such as heavy lifting) or to maintain control of equipment or tools
- Repetition—performing the same motion or series of motions continually or frequently
- Awkward postures—assuming positions that place stress on the body, such as reaching above shoulder height, kneeling, squatting, leaning over a bed, or twisting the torso while lifting[14]

A number of disorders can arise in workers with excessive exposure to these risk factors. Collectively referred to as musculoskeletal disorder (MSD), these conditions consist of low back pain, sciatica, rotator cuff injuries, epicondylitis, and carpal tunnel syndrome.[15] Early indications of MSD can include persistent pain, restriction of joint movement, or soft tissue swelling.[16]

Some MSDs can develop over time, and others may result in the midst of a procedure such as a single heavy lift. MSDs also may be related to genetic causes, gender, age, and other factors. Finally, there is evidence that reports of MSDs may be linked to certain psychosocial factors such as job dissatisfaction, monotonous work, and limited job control.

Providing an alternative to manual care recipient lifting is the primary goal of an

FIGURE 4-2

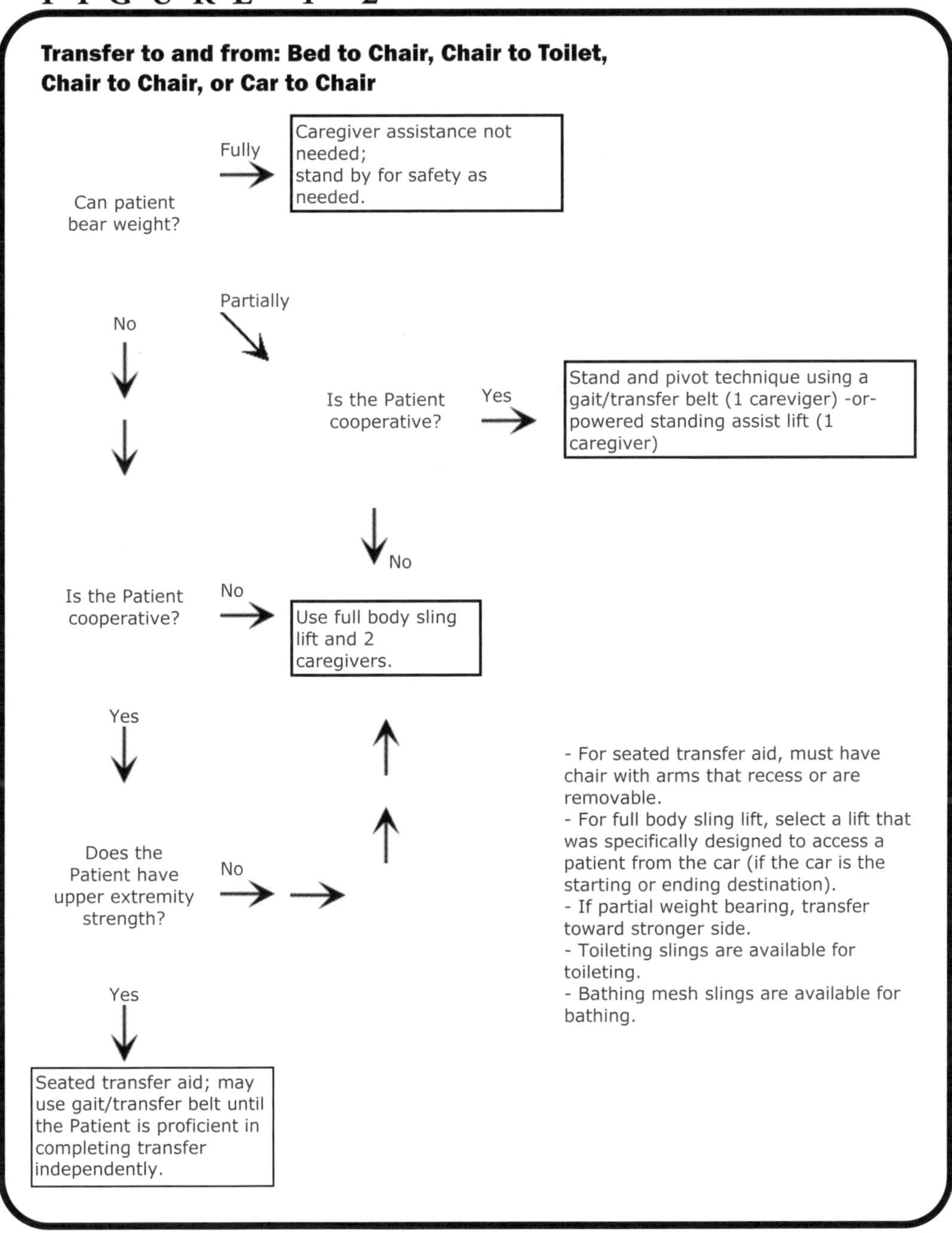

ergonomics process in the health care setting. OSHA recommends that manual lifting of care recipients be minimized in all cases and eliminated when feasible. OSHA further recommends that employers develop a process for systematically addressing ergonomics issues in their facilities and incorporate this process into an overall program to recognize and prevent occupational safety and health hazards. This process, according to OSHA, should be tailored

FIGURE 4-3

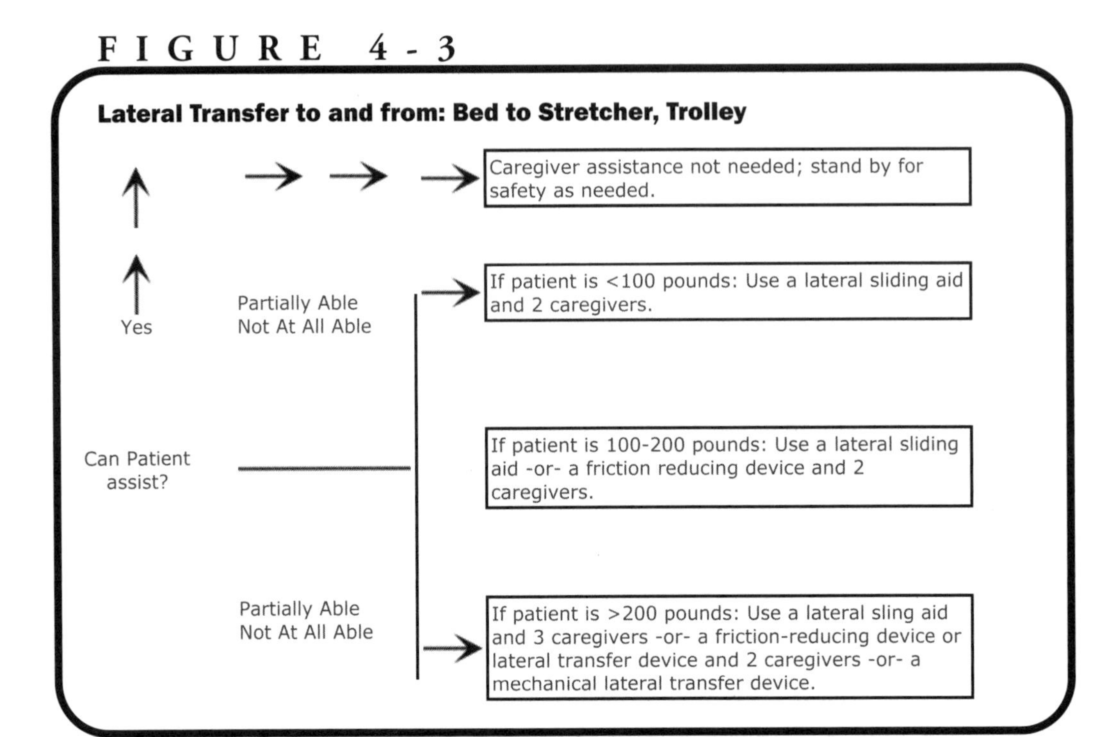

FIGURE 4-4

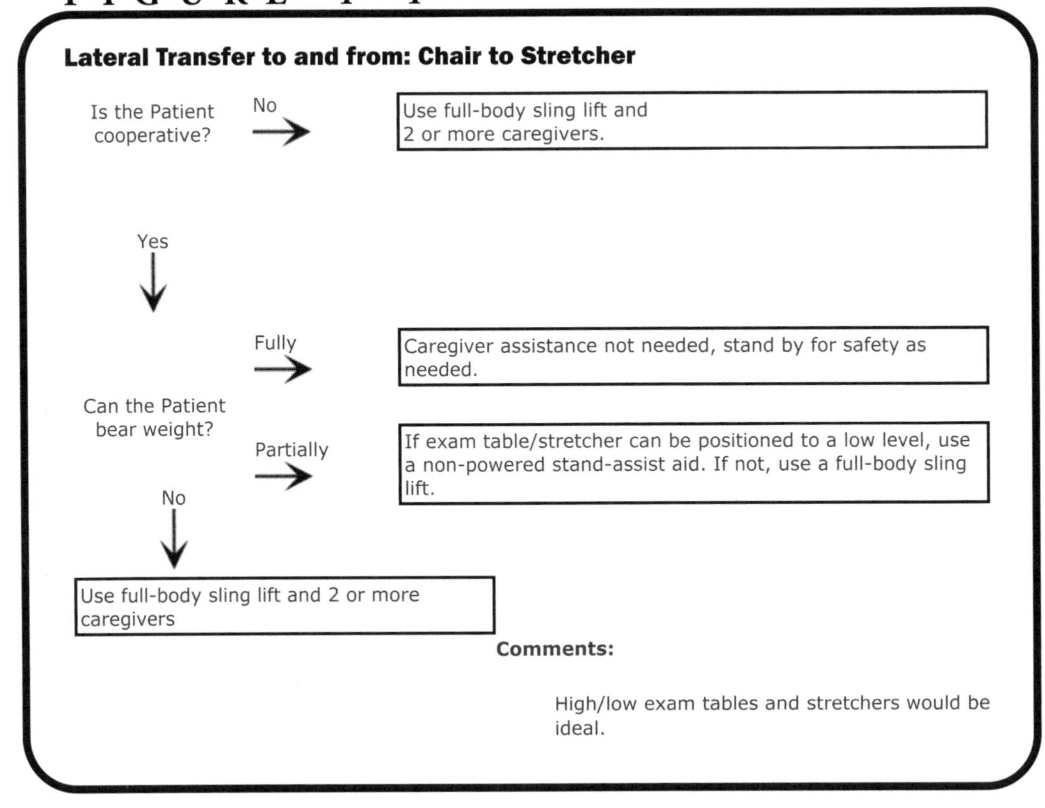

FIGURE 4-5

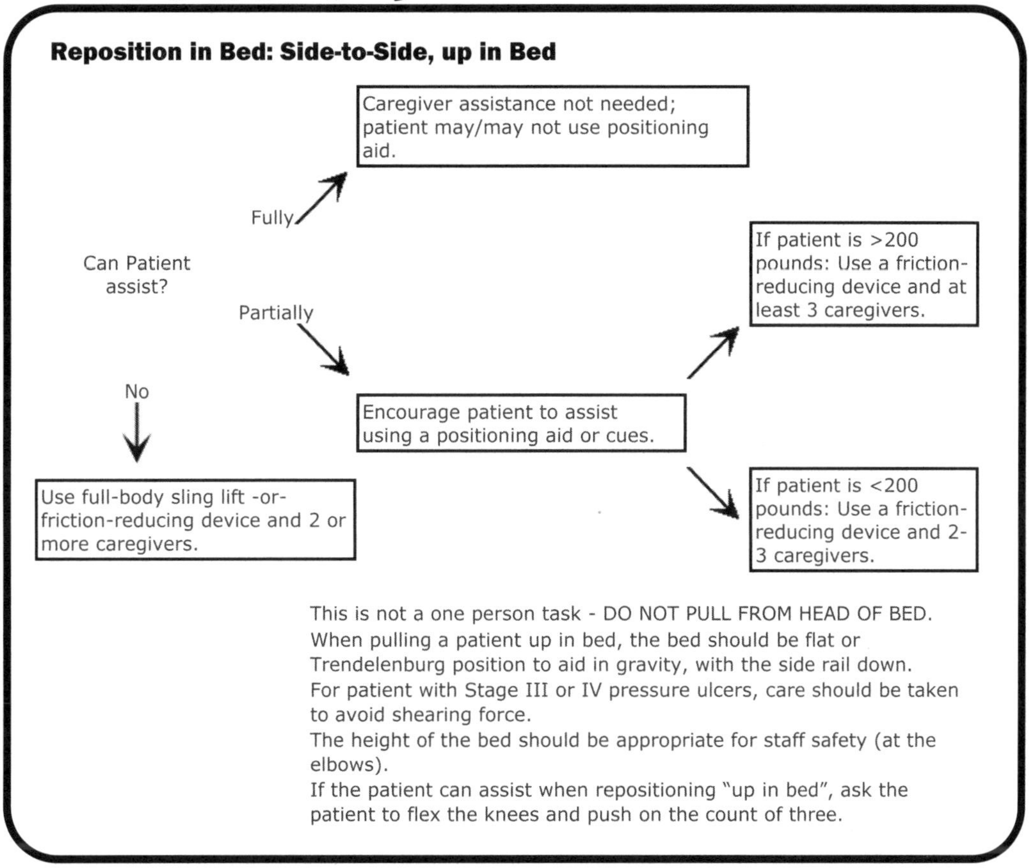

Reposition in Bed: Side-to-Side, up in Bed

Can Patient assist?

Fully → Caregiver assistance not needed; patient may/may not use positioning aid.

Partially → Encourage patient to assist using a positioning aid or cues.

→ If patient is >200 pounds: Use a friction-reducing device and at least 3 caregivers.

→ If patient is <200 pounds: Use a friction-reducing device and 2-3 caregivers.

No → Use full-body sling lift -or- friction-reducing device and 2 or more caregivers.

This is not a one person task - DO NOT PULL FROM HEAD OF BED.
When pulling a patient up in bed, the bed should be flat or Trendelenburg position to aid in gravity, with the side rail down.
For patient with Stage III or IV pressure ulcers, care should be taken to avoid shearing force.
The height of the bed should be appropriate for staff safety (at the elbows).
If the patient can assist when repositioning "up in bed", ask the patient to flex the knees and push on the count of three.

to fit the characteristics of the individual facility.

OSHA has suggested that nursing homes consider the steps outlined in Sidebar 4-3, page 102, in implementing an effective ergonomics process. These steps also relate to other health care settings.

Interventions That Maintain an Individualized Approach

No two care recipients are the same. Fall reduction can be effective, and approaches to intervention should be determined by the specific needs and wishes of each care recipient.

Care plans may involve addressing factors inherent to the individual care recipient, to the environment, or to both. For example, if residents are incontinent and nonambulatory (resident characteristics), placing them on regular toileting schedules can help prevent them from trying to get up on their own to go to the bathroom (staff process and training-environmental factor). Because falling can be due to an adverse drug reaction, an individualized drug regimen review is also critical.

Monitoring the care plan must also be individualized. If the care recipient is given newer shoes to help with walking, for example, staff should check the shoes in the first few days to assure that they are not too loose (a fall risk), or too tight (a pressure ulcer risk).

Communication is key in providing individualized care. Throughout the assessment, evaluation, care planning, and monitoring process, staff must consistently exchange information.

FIGURE 4-6

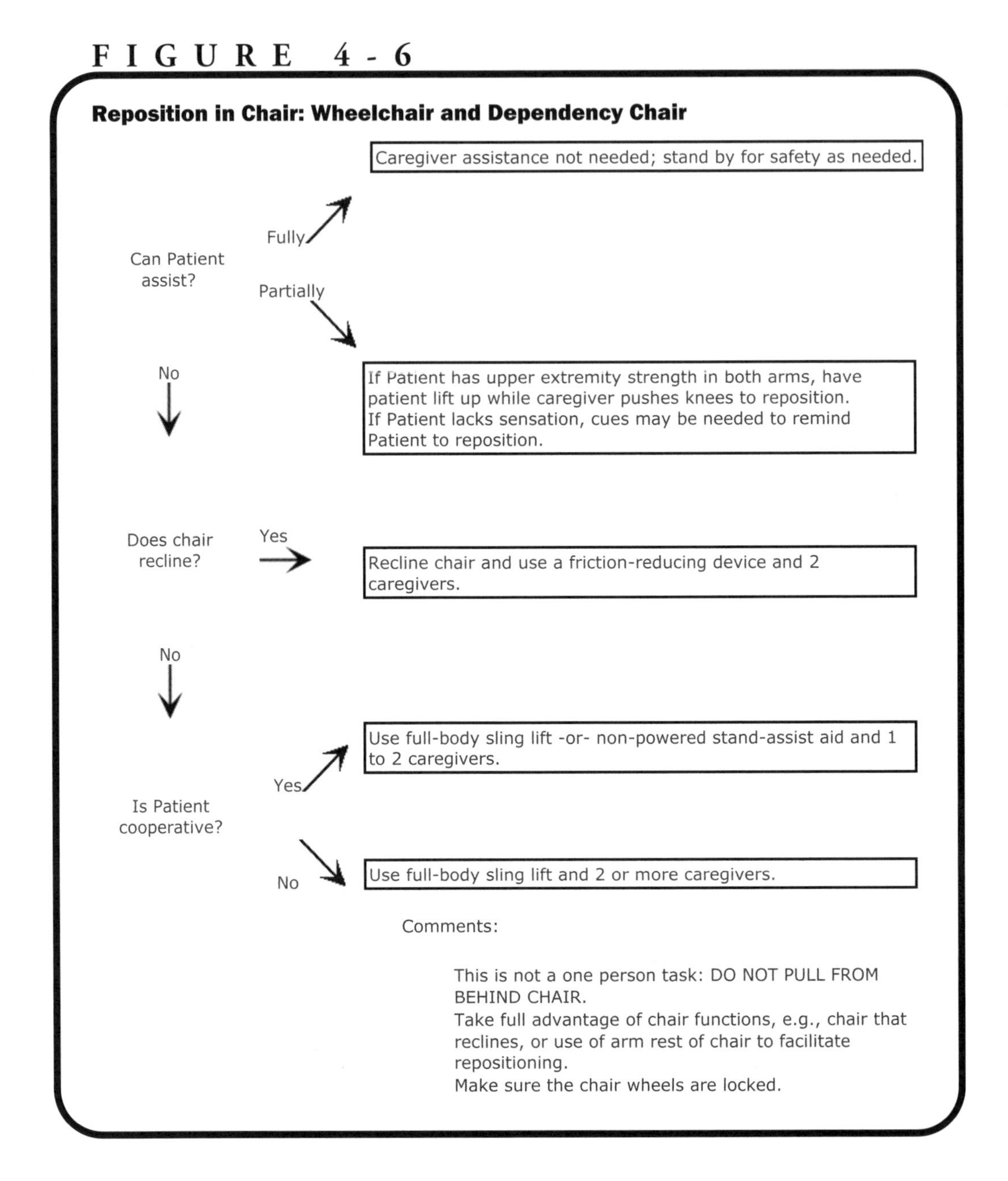

Each proposed workup or intervention must be weighed for its risks and benefits to a specific care recipient. For example, an end-stage care recipient with dementia may not benefit from being transferred to a hospital or other facility for a CT scan and invasive testing. However, for a healthier ambulatory resident, such testing may make sense.

In the report by Janice Morse, the researcher warns that "carte blanche application of protective or prevention policies may increase fall risk or risk of injury to some patients."

Interventions Supported by Research and Decision Making

Effective fall risk assessment tools empower

FIGURE 4-7

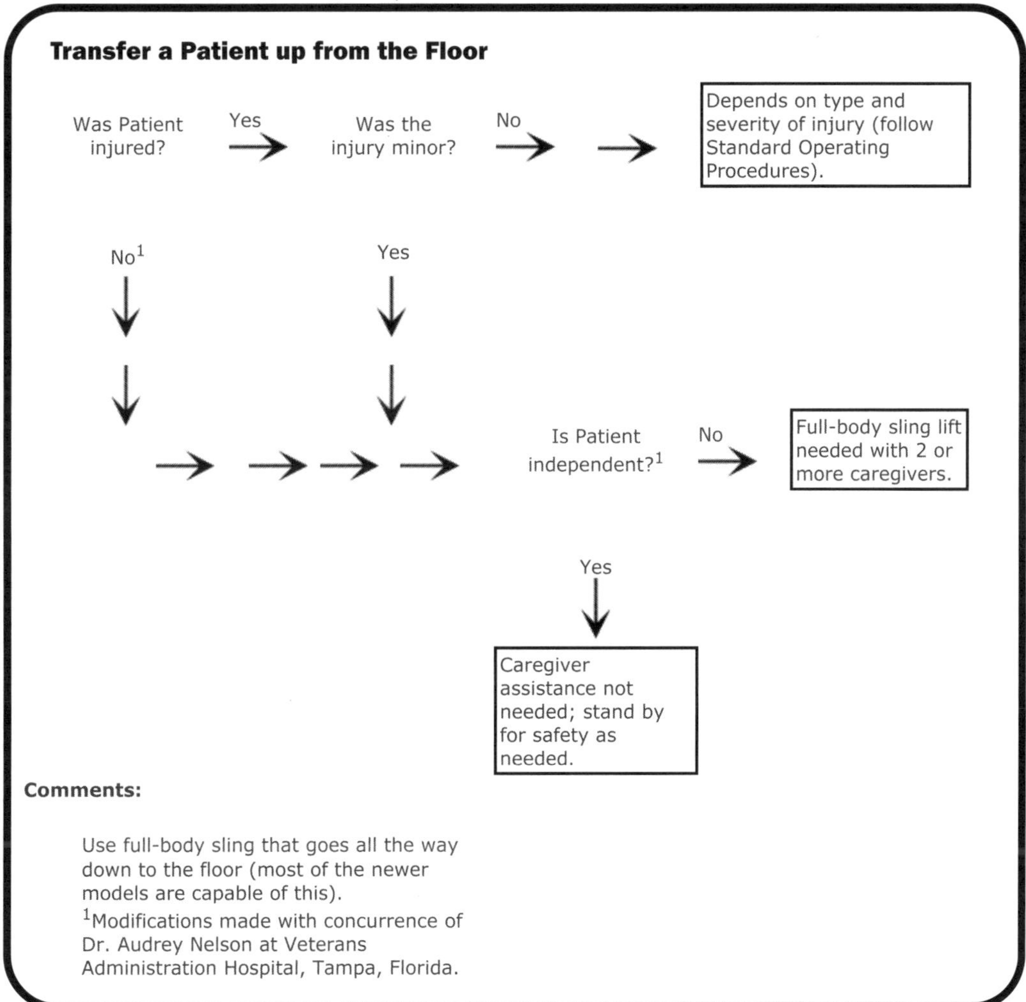

medical experts to make sound decisions about intervention. Based on the results of assessments, health care professionals use their clinical knowledge and judgment in applying the general principles and specific recommendations to the care management of individual care recipients. Decisions to adopt any particular recommendation must be made by the practitioner in light of available evidence and resources.

Many of the intervention decisions made by medical staff should come from literature obtained during the research phase of a plan to develop a fall reduction program. This includes systematic reviews and meta-analyses, randomized trials, controlled before-and-after studies, case-control studies and cohort studies with outcomes involving data related to fall risk or fall reduction, and articles that provide epidemiological or other background information.

The expert knowledge and experience of staff and fall team members also reinforces the search strategy. It is important to identify and synthesize relevant published evidence to allow recommendations to be evidence-based, whenever possible. The AGS Panel on Falls

SIDEBAR 4-3

Steps for Implementing an Effective Ergonomics Process

Provide Management Support

Strong support by management creates the best opportunity for success. OSHA recommends that employers develop clear goals, assign responsibilities to designated staff members to achieve those goals, provide necessary resources, and ensure that assigned responsibilities are fulfilled. Providing a safe and healthy workplace requires a sustained effort, allocation of resources, and frequent follow-up that can be achieved only through the active support of management.

Involve Employees

Employees are a vital source of information about hazards in their workplace. Their involvement adds problem-solving capabilities and hazard identification assistance, enhances worker motivation and job satisfaction, and leads to greater acceptance when changes are made in the workplace. Employees can do the following:

- Submit suggestions or concerns.
- Discuss the workplace and work methods.
- Participate in the design of work, equipment, procedures, and training.
- Evaluate equipment.
- Respond to employee surveys.
- Participate in task groups with responsibility for ergonomics.
- Participate in developing the nursing home's ergonomics process.

Identify Problems

Nursing homes can more successfully recognize problems by establishing systematic methods for identifying ergonomic concerns in their workplace. Information about where problems or potential problems may occur in nursing homes can be obtained from a variety of sources, including OSHA 300 and 301 injury and illness information, reports of workers' compensation claims, accident and near-miss investigation reports, insurance company reports, employee interviews, employee surveys, and reviews and observations of workplace conditions. After information is obtained, it can be used to identify and evaluate elements of jobs that are associated with problems.

Implement Solutions

When problems related to ergonomics are identified, suitable options can then be selected and implemented to eliminate hazards. Effective solutions usually involve workplace modifications that eliminate hazards and improve the work environment. These changes usually include the use of equipment, work practices, or both. When choosing methods for lifting and repositioning care recipients, individual factors should be taken into account. Such factors include the care recipient's rehabilitation plan, the need to restore the care recipient's functional abilities, medical contraindications, emergency situations, and care recipient dignity and rights.

(continued)

SIDEBAR 4-3 (continued)

Address Reports of Injuries

Even in organizations with effective safety and health programs, injuries and illnesses may occur. Work-related musculoskeletal disorders (MSDs) should be managed in the same manner and under the same process as any other occupational injury or illness. As with many injuries and illnesses, employers and employees can benefit from early reporting of MSDs. Early diagnosis and intervention, including alternative duty programs, are particularly important in order to limit the severity of injury, improve the effectiveness of treatment, minimize the likelihood of disability or permanent damage, and reduce the amount of associated workers' compensation claims and costs. OSHA's injury and illness recording and reporting regulation (29 CFR 1904) requires employers to keep records of work-related injuries and illnesses. These reports can help the nursing home identify problem areas and evaluate ergonomic efforts. Employees may not be discriminated against for reporting a work-related injury or illness.

Provide Training

Training is necessary to ensure that employees and managers can recognize potential ergonomic issues in the workplace and understand measures that are available to minimize the risk of injury. Ergonomic training can be integrated into general training on performance requirements and job practices. Effective training covers the problems found in each employee's job.

Evaluate Ergonomics Efforts

Nursing homes should evaluate the effectiveness of their ergonomics efforts and follow up on unresolved problems. Evaluation helps sustain the effort to reduce injuries and illnesses, track whether or not ergonomic solutions are working, identify new problems, and show areas where further improvement is needed. Evaluation and follow-up are central to continuous improvement and long-term success. When solutions are introduced, OSHA recommends that employers ensure that they are effective. Various indicators (for example, OSHA 300 and 301 information data and workers' compensation reports) can provide useful empirical data at this stage, as can other techniques such as employee interviews. For example, after introducing a new lift at a nursing home, the employer should follow up by talking with employees to ensure that the problem has been adequately addressed. In addition, interviews provide a mechanism for ensuring that the solution is not only in place, but is being used properly. The same methods that are used to identify problems, in many cases, can also be used for evaluation.

Prevention provides an example of one grading criteria in Sidebar 4-4, page 104.

The grading criteria distinguish between category of evidence and strength of the associated recommendation. It is possible to have methodologically sound (Class I) evidence about an area of practice that is clinically irrelevant or has such a small effect that it is of little practical importance and would, therefore, attract a lower strength of recommendation. More commonly, a statement of evidence would cover only one part of an area in which a recommendation has to be made or would cover it in a way that conflicted with other evidence. Therefore, to produce comprehensive recommendations, the health care organization may have to extrapolate from the available evidence. This may lead to weaker levels of recommendation (B, C, or D) based on Class I evidence statements.

Inevitably, this is a subjective process. It is

SIDEBAR 4-4

Grading Criteria

Categories of Evidence

Class I: Evidence from at least one randomized controlled trial or a meta-analysis of randomized controlled trials

Class II: Evidence from at least one controlled study without randomization or evidence from at least one other type of quasi-experimental study

Class III: Evidence from nonexperimental studies such as comparative studies, correlation studies, and case-control studies

Class IV: Evidence from expert committee reports or opinions and/or clinical experience of respected authorities

Strength of Recommendation

A: Directly based on Class I evidence

B: Directly based on Class II evidence or extrapolated recommendation from Class I evidence

C: Directly based on Class III evidence or extrapolated recommendation from Class I or II evidence

D: Directly based on Class IV evidence or extrapolated recommendation from Class I, II, or III evidence[17]

accepted that there will be areas without evidence where recommendations should be made, and that consensus will be required to address such areas. Where there is not sufficient evidence to make recommendations, it is important that unanswered research questions be documented in fall reduction reports.

According to the AGS Panel, risk factors identified in an assessment may be modifiable (such as muscle weakness, medication side effect, or hypotension) or nonmodifiable (such as hemiplegia or blindness). However, knowledge of all risk factors is important for treatment planning. Essential components of the fall-related care recipient assessment should be identified whenever possible from successful controlled trials of fall reduction interventions. The justification for assessment to identify a specific risk factor is strongest when successful treatment or other risk-reduction strategies have been explicitly based on this specific risk factor.

In some cases, the link between identified risk factors and the content of interventions is not clear. When conclusive data on the importance of specific aspects of the assessment (either to prediction of falls or to responsiveness of these risks factors to the intervention) are not available, consensus should be sought.

Collecting and Using Data in Developing Interventions

After implementing intervention strategies based on results from a comprehensive fall risk assessment, the accomplishments of a successful fall reduction program have only begun. In recognizing that fall risk is not static and can change quickly and frequently in any health care setting, health care organizations must be vigilant in the collection of further data that can contribute to more-focused care recipient intervention strategies.

Staff should be prepared to collect and consider care recipient data as part of an ongoing effort to improve the reduction plan. As part of a pilot program, teams may conduct retrospective chart reviews using an audit tool to look at all care recipients who have fallen, and an equal random sample of care recipients who have not yet experienced a fall. Though it has often gone underutilized, data collected from care recipients without a fall can be quite beneficial in determining whether measures implemented as part of the pilot were helpful in reducing falls.

Data gathered from a pilot program can, of course, help hone strategies to be tested and ultimately chosen as best practices to be implemented organizationwide. Additional chart review might also determine whether the documentation of fall risk and postfall are focused, uniform, and consistent across the organization.

Unit-specific data can reveal different information regarding each population's risk factors. For example, gait impairment may be revealed to be higher in the surgical care recipient population than the psychiatric care recipient population. If the majority of care recipients who fell in the surgical unit tended to fall as they were getting up from bed, usually to use the toilet, and most of the care recipients who fell on the psychiatric unit did so while ambulating down the hallway, the surgical unit can emphasize toileting issues while the psychiatric unit focuses on ambulation issues.

Unit-specific data can be most valuable because they enable units to tailor their improvements to their care recipient populations. Important fall data, which should be broken out into individual units as well as housewide, should be reviewed monthly, quarterly, and annually. The quality department can trend the data quarterly and provide them to staff accordingly.

In transitional care units (TCUs), geriatric units, and long term care facilities, nearly every care recipient meets the criteria of being at high risk of falls. The case study in Example 4-1 looks at the process of developing a unit-specific fall reduction program.

Consistent Documentation in the Intervention Process

To make both individual and global changes that result in a reduction of resident falls and injuries, a health organization's fall reduction

EXAMPLE 4-1

Developing a Unit-Specific Fall Reduction Program

Though an extensive amount of literature addresses the significance of patient falls and mechanisms to identify those at high risk, much less has been written regarding units in which nearly every patient fits the high-risk category. In addition, little information describes specific interventions designed to protect at-risk patients. In response to a record number of falls in the transitional care unit (TCU) at an acute care facility, an interdisciplinary team was developed to review patient falls, design a unit-specific fall reduction program, and begin its implementation. In the subsequent six quarters, the number of patient falls was reduced by 57%.

In the fourth quarter, the TCU of an urban 688-bed acute care facility encountered its highest number of patient falls ever recorded. The unit provided care to Medicare patients who were, by definition, either older than 65 years or persons with a disability. The admission criteria to

(continued)

EXAMPLE 4-1 (continued)

the unit placed greater than 90% of these patients at high risk for falls according to the hospital's fall assessment tool. A retrospective review of each fall occurring in the fourth quarter was conducted to determine proximate and distal causes. This review formed the foundation for the initial fall reduction program.

In addition, each fall that occurred from that quarter onward was similarly reviewed. New interventions were added after each review to reduce the risk of similar falls occurring in the future. This resulted in the development of fall reduction strategies specific to the unit and its patient population.

Process

To design the fall reduction program, the TCU utilized a FOCUS-PDCA approach (**F**ind an improvement opportunity, **O**rganize a team that knows the process, **C**larify current knowledge of the process, **U**ncover root cause of the process variation, **S**tart the improvement by implementing a **P**lan of action. **D**o tests and collect data, **C**heck the results, **A**ct). The first step—find a problem to improve—appeared self-evident. The unit's fall index, defined as the number of falls per 1,000 patient days, was 9.2. Hospital staff utilized Henrich's definition of a patient fall as "any unanticipated change in body position in a downward motion that may or may not result in physical injury."

The second process step involved the organization of an interdisciplinary team. The importance of utilizing a multidisciplinary approach is to comprehensively address the multifactorial cause of falls in older persons. In addition, the multidisciplinary nature of patient care on the unit demanded the development of an equally diverse problem-solving team.

Clarification of the problem involved a review of staffing patterns and the identification of characteristics of the patient population that increased risk for falls. Although staffing patterns were believed to be adequate, a review of patterns in TCUs across the country was conducted. The review indicated that this TCU's hours per patient day exceeded the mean for similar units. Furthermore, a comprehensive review of occurrence reports, chart data, and staff interview data regarding patient falls revealed several potential contributing factors to falls, such as the following:

- Recent changes in levels of independence
- Belief that asking for assistance bothers staff
- Slow adaptation to environmental changes
- Complex medication regimen and/or polypharmacy
- Short-term memory changes
- Poor impulse control
- Sensory changes (for example, visual, auditory, balance, awareness of elimination needs)
- Fine motor changes
- Communication difficulties

The aforementioned findings are consistent with the types of falls identified as extrinsic (for example, related to environmental factors), iatrogenic (for example, related to treatment

(continued)

EXAMPLE 4-1 (continued)

factors), and intrinsic (for example, related to host factors). Further data analysis also revealed the following trends:

- Patients forgot to call for assistance.
- Patients did not want to bother the staff.
- Some falls occurred when patients were monitored by non-nursing disciplines (for example, physical therapy staff, radiology staff, family members).
- Falls occurred more frequently during change of shift.
- Falls occurred while patients were attempting to ambulate to the bathroom.
- Some residents experienced multiple falls.

After each occurrence report was analyzed, a strategy was developed for that specific type of fall, and that strategy was included in the unit's safety program. Interventions were designed to increase patient and staff awareness and provide increased staff supervision. Staff were educated via monthly meetings, e-mail, impromptu meetings, falls committee meetings, new staff orientation, and meetings with patients and families.

Interventions

A review of the literature revealed little data on specific interventions designed to reduce falls among older adults. The interdisciplinary team created and developed all tools, and additional interventions were added to the safety program as these interventions were generated.

To remind patients to ask for assistance when getting out of bed, yellow road sign–shaped caution signs were created and posted in each patient room. These signs stated, "Caution! Ask for assistance whenever getting up! Please help prevent falls and fall-related injuries." These signs were also illustrated with the representation of a stick figure slipping and falling.

In addition, a "safety with dignity" flier was developed and reviewed with patients. This flier acknowledged the loss of control patients experience and their desire for independence. The flier addressed the changes in environment, medications, and functional ability that increase patients' risk of falling. Patients were assured that they were not bothering staff by asking for staff assistance. The flier included safety tips and the telephone number of the nurses' station in case the patient misplaced the call light. Finally, the flier included a description of actions to take, should a patient actually fall.

Although all geriatric patients may be identified as being at high risk for falls, it is essential to recognize patients at the greatest risk. Upon review of patient falls within the unit, certain criteria emerged that help identify those at very high risk. These criteria included the following:

- Patients who demonstrated poor impulse control
- Patients with short-term memory deficits
- Patients who were unable to demonstrate use of the call light
- Patients who had experienced previous falls

The last criterion was also consistent with Patrick and Blodget's findings that a history of previous falls significantly increased a patient's risk of subsequent falls.

(continued)

EXAMPLE 4-1 (continued)

To increase both family and staff awareness of patients who are at very high risk for falls, the Guardian Program was created. In essence, the program implemented surveillance and clear delineation of responsibility. The staff member responsible for ensuring a high-risk patient's safety wore a TCU Guardian badge illustrated with an angel. When someone else assumed responsibility for the patient (for example, a family member, physical therapy staff, or radiology staff), the badge was passed on. This clearly identified the person safeguarding the patient and reinforced responsibility for the specific patient's safety. When the Guardian Program was implemented with patients, the program was discussed with the patient and family, and printed material describing the program was provided.

Unfortunately, patients identified at very high risk for falls did not always have the available family or staff required to participate in the Guardian Program. In these cases, in addition to increasing the frequency of visual checks by staff, the use of a bed alarm helped staff respond to patients attempting to get out of bed without assistance. If a patient set off the alarm continually by constant efforts to get out of bed, a sitter was provided.

Additional interventions were also developed to increase staff awareness of patient safety. When patients from acute care hospital units were received, previous falls were not always mentioned. The forms used for receiving reports on new admissions were modified to include a fall history component. After patients were admitted to the TCU, fall risk was included in every shift-to-shift report. Finally, a large dry-erase calendar was posted in the employee break room. Every fall for the month was documented on the calendar, and the number of falls for each month of the previous year was also recorded. In this way, staff members could visualize the progress they were making toward their goal.

Analysis of occurrence reports identified a tendency of patients to fall at the change of shift. The TCU nursing staff received shift-to-shift reports in the activity room, which decreased the number of staff available to meet patient needs during this time. Walking rounds were implemented as the means to give and receive shift-to-shift reports. This action effectively doubled the number of staff available to provide patient care at change of shift.

To reduce bathroom-related falls, staff offered toileting assistance every two hours while patients were awake. Although this decreased daytime falls, patients often fell when they awoke early in the morning and attempted to go to the bathroom without assistance. Staff routinely woke confused patients between 5:30 A.M. and 7:00 A.M. and offered toileting assistance. Nurses reported that this intervention contributed most significantly to reducing the total number of patient falls.

If patients did experience a fall, three additional interventions were implemented. The interdisciplinary team immediately reviewed the circumstances surrounding the fall and identified strategies that could have possibly reduced the risk of it occurring. The manager reviewed this report, and the unit safety program was modified, if necessary, or staff members were educated or counseled as needed. A family conference was held to discuss the fall and develop a patient-focused fall reduction plan. Families were often able to provide information

(continued)

EXAMPLE 4-1 (continued)

relating to the following:

- Identification of covert confusion not apparent to staff members
- Identification of patient's individual elimination patterns
- Description of patient-specific symptoms of agitation

Tools

In addition to the yellow caution signs, the Guardian Program badges and handout, and the "safety with dignity" flier, several other tools were utilized. The facility occurrence reports identified the patient and staff involved in a patient fall and briefly described the circumstances. The Falls Interdisciplinary Conference form included in the same information, documented when toileting assistance was last offered and included suggestions to reduce falls of a similar nature. The Quality Care/Patient Fall Assessment form was used throughout the hospital to evaluate falls and included information such as patient risk for fall, previous fall history, classification of patient outcome (for example, level of injury), fall strategies already in place, patient use of call light, and circumstances of fall.

Challenges

As the safety plan was implemented, several problems were identified and the plans were modified as needed. Initially, the case manager who met with every new admission provided the "safety with dignity" flier. Unfortunately, some patients were admitted on the weekend and fell before the case manager met with them on Monday. To avoid this problem, the safety with dignity information was included in the patient admission packet and reviewed by nursing staff upon unit admission.

Although the initial safety plan included members of an interdisciplinary team, not all modifications were disseminated to all disciplines. Fortunately, the ancillary staff in the TCU were typically constant, so any changes to the plan were forwarded to the therapies manager who educated the ancillary staff.

Some patient falls occurred because new staff were unaware of the safety program. To reduce falls of this type, the safety program was included in the unit-specific new employee orientation.

Results

Hospital staff utilized the fall index to quantify and normalize patient falls. This value is defined as the number of patient falls per month divided by total patient days multiplied by 1,000. The fall index peaked in the fourth quarter of 1998 at 9.32 falls. At this point, the initial fall reduction plan was implemented; interventions were added during the next three quarters. The fall index dropped from 9.32 to 6.09 by the first quarter of 1999, representing a reduction of 35%. The index continued to decrease, and by the fourth quarter of 1999, one year after program implementation, the fall index of 4.28 represented a reduction of 54%. The fall index remained below 5.0 for the next two quarters, with a low index of 4.01, or 57% below the initial index.

(continued)

EXAMPLE 4-1 (continued)

During the time frame that the falls reduction program was developed and implemented, the length of stay in the unit decreased by 6.9%. Although a relationship between program implementation and reduced length of stay (LOS) cannot be proven at this point, a likely explanation is that the program reduced falls and associated injuries. In turn, reduction in fall-related injuries reduced the LOS.

This fall reduction program was developed in response to a serious problem, and the interventions were added incrementally. Although the program significantly reduced falls, it does not constitute rigorous research. In particular, because this program was developed at the only TCU in the area, it was not possible to utilize a control group. However, the fall reduction program could be applied to any acute or long term care setting serving a geriatric population. The use of a control group in future research would strengthen the significance of the results.

Conclusion

Although this program did not meet criteria characterizing research, the results are nevertheless significant to the TCU patients and hospital staff. The other units in the hospital were successfully reducing the risk of falls using an existing housewide fall reduction program. However, the record number of falls reported in 1998 makes it clear that the geriatric housewide plan did not meet the needs of the TCU patients. The results of the TCU fall reduction program demonstrate the importance of reviewing and applying data collected on specific populations. Using the figure of $22,000 per fall cited by Haumschild et al.—who quantified the costs associated with patient falls—the reduction of falls from 9.32 to 4.02 in the TCU represents an average monthly savings of $116,600. If similar results are obtained throughout the country, annual fall-related costs could decrease from $406,000,000 to $174,580,000, and 1,026 lives could be saved. Finally, the decreased length of stay in TCU concurrent with the fall reduction program allowed patients to rejoin their families sooner.

Although some of the techniques developed may prove useful in other settings, the most significant result of this study is the process utilized to apply performance improvement data to specific populations. The process could be applied to any area of concern.

In summary, although patients fall for a variety of reasons, using performance improvement data specific to staff and patient populations could direct the development of a successful fall reduction program.[18]

program relies on forms, policies, and procedures that consistently track falls and identify commonalities.

Although health care organizations have policies and procedures in place describing how to report accidents and incidents, some do not have a standard way to classify, investigate, or track falls. Others may not have a common way to categorize injuries that result from falls or keep track of those who fall, making it difficult to analyze fall information in order to make sound adjustments to the care of the recipient.

In reviewing forms and policies, it is beneficial to review literature to help determine what is missing and to revise current forms and policies or create new ones as needed. When there

FIGURE 4-8

Accident/Incident Investigation

Resident name	Age	Type of Incident	Type of Injury

Classification of Injury			
0-No injury	1-Minor	2-Moderate	3-Major

Activity at Time of Incident		
1-Ambulating independently	2-Ambulating with walker	3-Ambulating with cane/crutches
4-Ambulating with staff/family	5-Attempting to stand or transfer	6-Getting out of bed
7-Attempting to get out of bed	8-Reaching or bending	9-Attempting to sit

Medications Within 24 Hours of Incident					
1-Narcotics	2-Tranquilizers	3-Antidepressants	4-Antipsychotics	5-Sedatives	
6-Anticonvulsants	7-Diuretics	8-Non-narcotic analgesics	9-Antihypertensives	10-Anticoagulants	11-Vasodilators

Change in Medication Regimen in Last 72 Hours

Functional/Mental Status at Time of Incident			
1-Alert, oriented in all spheres	2-Awake, confused	3-Awake, agitated, confused	4-Oriented all spheres, drowsy
5-Drowsy, confused	6-Blind	7-Deaf	

History of Falls or Other Incidents

Medical Condition Predisposing to Falls

Environmental Factors		
1-Floors wet/slippery	2-Poor lighting/glare	3-Bedrails up
4-Wheelchair brakes working	5-Walker/cane without tips	6-No footwear/inappropriate footwear

Analysis of Findings

Signature____________________ Date ___________ ☐ CP Reviewed

Editor's note: This form may or may not apply to the services your organization provides. Rather than using it verbatim, use it as a reference and as a starting point to develop your own document.

is no clear classification of injuries, organizations may tend to avoid investigating those with no injury. All falls should be investigated

Every month, a nursing director might review all incident and investigation reports, looking for common factors such as medications being taken by the care recipient, the care recipient's environment, or the care recipient's activity at the time of the fall. Based on these investigations, staff are better equipped to address the care recipient's immediate needs and to take measures that might reduce the risk of a future fall, such as adjusting the care recipient's environment or recommending physical therapy.

These data should also be reviewed with the medical director and the interdisciplinary team to help identify more global issues that could be addressed. For example, if several residents fell from wheelchairs during transfer, the maintenance department should inspect all wheelchairs for defects. At the same time, reeducation of staff and residents on the importance of locking wheels during transfer might also be effective.

Based on incident and investigation reports, organizations can create a monthly summary report for the quality improvement team. Consistency in forms and data collection is crucial to helping identify and address problems.

The case study in Example 4-2 on page 112

outlines the ways in which one health care organization's fall team looked to evidence-based approaches, and a quality improvement and incentive plan, in setting measurable new goals for its fall reduction program.

Institutional Support for Interventions

Morse has strongly suggested that successful intervention strategies require as much support from the health care institution as from its staff. "A fall reduction program is not simply an 'add on'—something that staff can simply add to their work load without incurring any additional costs—implementation must be planned and systematic and include staff training," she says in the previously mentioned report: "Enhancing the Safety of Hospitalization by Reducing Patient Falls."

Intervention programs should get the con-

EXAMPLE 4-2

Fall Reduction Program Yields Quick Results

In December 2002, Northeast Health System (NHS), in Beverly, Massachusetts, launched a comprehensive fall reduction program at its two acute care hospitals, Addison Gilbert Hospital and Beverly Hospital. Immediately preceding the program's launch, a team composed of quality improvement staff, nursing leadership, and the care recipient safety committee reviewed the fall data from the two hospitals' nursing units and noticed an increase in the rate of falls, particularly in the rate of falls with injury. At about the same time, Blue Cross/Blue Shield of Massachusetts began a quality improvement incentive program and was seeking proposals for hospital/health system quality/patient safety initiatives. The timing could not have been better for the creation of a fall reduction project focused on the acute care population at NHS, utilizing the QI Project's Acute Care Indicator 13: *Documented Falls.*

According to Diane Dick, NHS assistant vice president of quality/case management, patient falls data have been reported, investigated, and trended for years. "This spike in volume and severity of falls was troubling, and it was clear that the entire falls program needed revising," says Dick.

The goal of NHS's falls reduction program is to decrease the number and severity of inpatient falls to be consistent with national and state means. To be most effective, however, the NHS team—composed of medical/surgical nursing leadership, performance improvement staff, staff nurses, representatives from the critical care unit, emergency department, obstetrics, physical therapy, education, and pharmacy—conducted a review of the literature and, utilizing an evidence-based approach, set a measurable goal for the program. The QI Project's aggregate mean rates for documented medical/surgical falls per 100 patient days for January through September 2002 ranged from 0.36 to 0.39. At NHS hospitals, the rate of falls per 100 patients ranged from 0.30 to 0.66. With this in mind, the NHS team's goal was to decrease the rate of falls per 100 patient days to below the projectwide mean rates by June 2003 and below .31 falls per 100 patient days by June 2004.

(continued)

EXAMPLE 4-2 (continued)

Remarkably, after the first six months of the project, as of June 30, 2003, the data showed a dramatic overall reduction in the rate of falls for the health system. In fact, for the first half of 2003, NHS's rate was below the projectwide mean rates. NHS had met and exceeded its 18-month goal in only 6 months.

Chart 4-1. Documented Falls

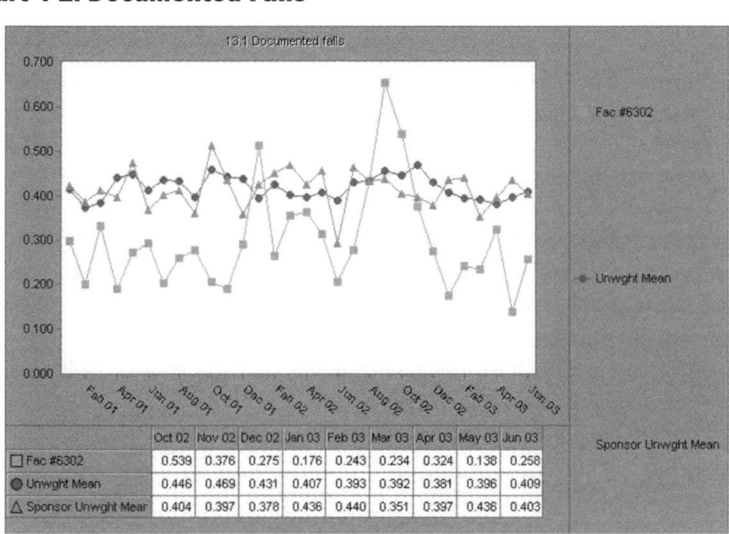

	Oct 02	Nov 02	Dec 02	Jan 03	Feb 03	Mar 03	Apr 03	May 03	Jun 03
□ Fac #6302	0.539	0.376	0.275	0.176	0.243	0.234	0.324	0.138	0.258
● Unwght Mean	0.446	0.469	0.431	0.407	0.393	0.392	0.381	0.396	0.409
△ Sponsor Unwght Mear	0.404	0.397	0.378	0.436	0.440	0.351	0.397	0.436	0.403

Note: Data points for mean rates between January 2002 and June 2003 are shown graphically for Northeast (facility) and the QI Project (sponsor); numerical values highlight the study period and portray the dramatic improvement.

How did NHS achieve this remarkable reduction in falls? Its multifaceted approach to implementing changes and interventions included the following:

- **Using a reliable and valid instrument to predict and identify prone-to-fall patients.** NHS developed a risk assessment tool, which is used to assess patients at admission and at each shift change. The assessment is based on the Morse Fall Scale and is recorded in an electronic log, along with the appropriate risk-reduction strategies and interventions associated with each patient's risk level. Nurse managers now receive daily reports of at-risk patients and post them on the units, and high-risk patients are identified with an easy-to-see gold star on the unit.
- **Developing a system to track incidence and type of falls institutionwide.** The team revised the fall report to include more information on the factors that contribute to falls. Additionally, an update to the administrative database allows better unit-specific information for trending and the ability to develop interventions that are appropriate to the patient population. Finally, the team established definitions for both fall and injury that could be used facilitywide.

(continued)

EXAMPLE 4-2 (continued)

- **Maintaining a safe environment.** The team worked with plant operations to examine potential environmental fall factors and performed checks on items such as beds, wheelchairs, walkers, handrail placement, and bathroom call bells. The fall reduction program coincided with the purchase of many new beds that were equipped with bed alarms.
- **Developing and targeting interventions for those likely to fall.** A multipronged approach, including administrative, direct care, environmental, and equipment initiatives, included identifying patients with a high-risk fall score by placing a gold star on the unit, then regularly toileting those patients, ensuring that they had adequate lighting at night, appropriately placing patients near the nursing station, and equipping those patients' beds and chairs with alarms.
- **Reducing the risk of those likely to fall.** To achieve this, NHS created a fall committee, and a clinical educator was assigned to provide ongoing fall education to staff and physicians. The committee conducts fall rounds, during which they provide direct education regarding current fall assessments. In addition, the educator is available to nursing units to conduct a fall reduction consult and recommend interventions.
- **Constantly monitoring patients who have fallen using a postfall protocol.** NHS developed an assessment and reporting flow sheet for nurses and physicians to provide standardized monitoring, treatment, and physician/family notification after a fall. The flow sheet outlines very concise responsibilities and steps for staff to follow after a patient experiences a fall.

NHS has made tremendous strides in reducing falls, but its work is yet to be completed. In addition to working to sustain its improvements, NHS wants to expand the scope of the fall program. While the initial focus was the medical/surgical areas, NHS is now customizing the assessment/treatment tools for use in the ambulatory and psychiatric settings. NHS is also working to create computer-based links between assessment and intervention—greatly enhancing the program's visibility with clinical staff. Other initiatives under way include implementing additional recommended environmental changes, expanding education beyond nursing to all ancillary departments, continued creation of fall reduction strategies by the multidisciplinary fall team, and testing new interventions such as chair alarms.

"Sharing success with all of our staff is particularly important," comments Dick. "We want our whole organization to know about and learn from the falls reduction program. To do this, we are creating posters for each unit showing the reduction in falls and are developing articles for placement in our organizational newsletter like the nursing newsletter."

According to Margaret Burns, nursing director for inpatient services, one of NHS's biggest ongoing challenges—one encountered during the early months of the fall reduction program—is staff education. "We underestimated both the time that it would take to educate the staff initially and the need for continuing education on the use of the assessment tool, interventions, documentation, and feedback from auditing," she says. "Now that we are expanding education beyond nursing, we are working to ensure that we have the resources necessary to meet the ongoing educational challenges."

The NHS team attributes the success of the program to its excellent nursing staff and team approach to patient care. Although NHS has seen dramatic improvements from the fall reduction program, patient falls will continue be one of its highest-priority safety issues.

tinual attention and cohesive support of colleagues from various disciplines, with each offering their specific expertise, wealth of knowledge, and professional commitment. As a team they should be empowered to go beyond the process of researching, planning, and implementing intervention strategies and be willing to add staff positions to ensure that all the pieces to carry out the plan are in place.

For example, Morse insists that appointing a clinical nurse specialist (CNS) who would be responsible for establishing and maintaining the fall reduction program is essential. The responsibilities of the CNS would include the following:

- Consistent use of the fall prediction instrument, the Morse Fall Scale (MFS). All nursing staff should be instructed in using the MFS. One of the responsibilities of the CNS will be to provide staff in-service education.
- Fall assessment of high-risk care recipients and care recipients who fall repeatedly. Care recipients who score at risk of falling must be individually assessed to identify appropriate fall protective care plans. Because these care plans are individualized (and often creative), the CNS will, over time, build a compendium of successful strategies.
- Coordination of the fall committee. The role of the multidisciplinary fall committee is to examine care recipients who are at very high risk of falling or have experienced repeated falls. Assessment may include a gait assessment and adjustment of medications, with the aim of reducing the care recipients' fall scores.
- Requisition, maintenance, and in-service of fall protective devices. Reducing accidental falls requires constant vigilance for hazards and continual upkeep of equipment.

Morse notes that the principles of institutional approaches for ensuring care recipient safety include establishing a system for monitoring care recipient falls, establishing a coordinated program for reducing care recipient falls, and ensuring adequate funding for fall protection.

These principles are also among the aspects that help measure the progress and success of a fall reduction program, which are outlined in further detail in the chapter ahead.

References

1. *NHPCO Insurance Update* 4:2, 2004.
2. Henkel G.: Beyond the MDS: Team approach to falls assessment, prevention, & management. *Caring for the Ages* 3:15–20, Apr. 2002.
3. Dimant J., et al.: Proceedings of NYOAS Best Practices Conference on Promotion of Mobility Independence in Long-Term Care Facilities, New York State Department of Health and Hunter/Mount Sinai Geriatric Education Center. *Caring for the Ages* 3:15–20, Apr. 2002.
4. Morse, J.M.: Enhancing the safety of hospitalization by reducing patient falls. *Am J Infect Control* 30:376–80, Jun. 2002.
5. National Center for Patient Safety (NCPS): VHA NCPS Falls Toolkit. May 2004. http://www.va.gov/ncps/SafetyTopics/fallstoolkit/notebook/index.html (accessed Feb. 9, 2005).
6. Morse J.M.: *Preventing Patient Falls.* Thousand Oaks, CA: Sage Publications, 1997.
7. Rubenstein, L.Z., Powers C., MacLean C.: Quality Indicators for the Management and Prevention of Falls and Mobility Problems in Vulnerable Elders (ACOVE). *Ann Intern Med* 135(pt. 2):686–693, Oct. 16, 2001.
8. Alexander N,B.: Gait disorders in older adults. *J Am Geritr Soc* 44:434–451, 1996. [PMID: 8636592]
9. Trueblood P.R., Rubenstein L.Z.: Assessment of instability and gait in elderly persons. *Compr Ther.* 1991;17:20–9. [PMID: 1742974].
10. Alexander N.B.: Gait disorders in older adults. *J Am Geritr Soc* 44:434–451, 1996. [PMID: 8636592].
11. Masdeu J.C., Sudarsky L., Wolfson L. (eds.): *Gait Disorders of Aging.* Philadelphia: Lippincott-Raven, 1997.
12. U.S. Department of Labor, Occupational Safety & Health Administration (OSHA): Ergonomics Guidelines for Nursing Homes. 2005. http://www.osha.gov/ergonomics/guidelines/nursinghome/final_nh_guidelines.html (accessed Feb. 12, 2005).
13. Garg A.: *Long-Term Effectiveness of "Zero-Lift Program" in Seven Nursing Homes and One Hospital.* Cincinnati: U.S. Department of Health and Human Services, Centers for Disease Control and Prevention, National Institution for Occupational Safety and Health. Aug. 1999 Contract No. U60/CCU512089-02. (Ex. 3-3).
14. Fragala G.: *Ergonomics: How to Contain On-the-Job Injuries in Health Care.* Oakbrook Terrace, IL: Joint Commission on Accreditation of Healthcare Organizations, 1996.
15. National Research Council and Institute of Medicine: *Musculoskeletal Disorders and the Workplace—Low Back and Upper Extremities.* National Academy of Sciences. Washington, DC: National Academy Press (Ex. 3-6), 2001.
16. Taylor, F.: *Cumulative Trauma Disorders: A Manual for MSDs of the Upper Limb.*, 1988.
17. AGS Panel on Falls Prevention. *JAGS* 49, May 2001.
18. Ward A., Candela L., Mahoney J.: Developing a unit-specific falls reduction program. *J Healthc Qual* 26:36–40, Mar./Apr. 2004.
19. Joint Commission Resources: Consistent documentation reduces resident falls. *Joint Commission: The Source* 1:8–9, Aug. 2003.

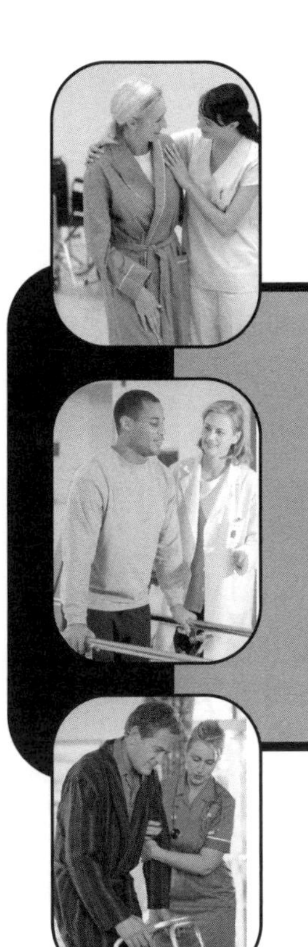

CHAPTER 5

Measuring Success of a Fall Reduction Program

The iatrogenic nation places patients at a risk of falling, injury, and death. It is our responsibility to provide protective and preventive interventions to minimize and eliminate this risk. Understanding the principles of fall interventions, and the role of and appropriate use of fall protective and preventive interventions—and implementing a comprehensive program that targets interventions appropriately and effectively—will meet the goal of providing safe care efficiently and at minimal cost.[1]

A health care organization cannot achieve its highest standards of appropriate and effective care without measuring its progress along the way. This chapter examines the ways in which health care organizations measure the effectiveness of a fall reduction program, and demonstrates the important role that proper application of data plays in an organization's efforts to reduce falls. It includes a review of Joint Commission standards designed to guide organizations in data collection and measurement, as well as examples of how proper performance evaluation can help improve and/or sustain a fall reduction program.

Necessary Steps Toward Measuring Program Effectiveness

Before measuring any goals in any setting, it is essential that these goals are clearly established and communicated from the very beginning. As for a fall reduction program, there are four basic steps to measuring the success of a program, as outlined in the Veterans Health Administration (VHA) National Center for Patient Safety (NCPS) Falls Toolkit.

Step One: Start at the Beginning

The first step is to define what you are reviewing. This involves going back to where you started.

For falls, you will need to develop a definition of a fall. As discussed in Chapter 1, literature offers a small variety of definitions from which many organizations customize to fit their program or facility. One frequently used definition of a fall is "a sudden, uncontrolled, unintentional downward displacement of the body to the ground or other object, excluding falls due to other purposeful actions."

When defining a fall, it is important to consider "unwitnessed falls" and different types of "near falls" such as trips or slips. The severity of injuries due to falls should also be defined and measured.[2] The VHA's standards for injury severity are as follows:

- 0 = None. No injury or disability.
- 1 = Minor injury (abrasion, bruise, minor laceration). Injuries are minor in nature, and if they do require any medical intervention, they do not extend the care recipients' hospital stay except for observation or to obtain laboratory and/or radiology results.
- 2 = Major injury (hip fracture, head trauma, arm fracture). Injuries that require medical or surgical intervention, increased hospital stay, or are disabling and/or disfiguring to a degree that the care recipient will have any degree of permanent lessened function or require surgical repair.
- 3 = Death[3]

Step Two: Deciding What to Measure and How

In determining what to measure and how, three different types of measurements are commonly used. They are outcome, process, and balancing measures.

Outcome measures help determine if the desired care recipient goal is being achieved. For example, are we reducing falls and injuries due to falls? With outcome measures, you can also examine organizational goals such as "Reduce severity of fall-related injury by 20%."

Process measures will tell you if you are implementing actions that are expected to lead to improvement. For example, you may choose to examine how many care recipients are assessed for fall risk, or the percentage of care recipients who fell and had all the indicated interventions in place. If you find that a high percentage of care recipients who fell did not have all of the indicated interventions implemented, you should likely focus on improving the use of fall reduction interventions. Another process measure is the percentage of staff trained in fall reduction.

Balancing measures are factors to monitor while you are improving one area to ensure that another area of care has not gotten worse. According to the VHA NCPS Toolkit, the measures you use should include the following rules:

1. Contains a numerator and denominator.
2. Specifies the time in which the information will be collected (for example, monthly, quarterly, or annually).
3. Specifies the measurement strategy (for example, observation, random checks of care recipient charts, or number of incident reports). Keep in mind that if you measure incident reports you are not measuring the actual number of incidents, but the level of reporting. This may skew your results.

Step Three: Collect Baseline Data

Once you have chosen your specific measures—such as fall rates or major injury rates—you will need to collect some baseline data. The baseline data are taken prior to the implementation of the program or a specific intervention. They are used to determine whether there is a change in your measures after the intervention is implemented. Keep in mind that you will need at least five or six baseline data points in order to ensure accurate data.

Step Four: Collection and Analysis of Data After Implementation

After implementing the program or specific intervention, you will need to keep measuring the data. You will require five or six data points after the implementation is complete to ensure accurate information. More information on this will be covered in the steps ahead.

Key Measures

The measures most often used in this process are fall rate and major injury rate. Most often, this information is best illustrated in a run chart. A run chart will be described in greater detail in the upcoming section on data analysis.

The *fall rate* is a measurement of risk. It tells you how many falls you can expect for every 1,000 bed days of care (BDOC).

Fall rate = (number of falls/BDOC) × 1,000 BDOC

BDOC tells you how many days care recipients were in beds. For example, if you have a census of 30 for 30 days, this is 900 BDOC. To obtain the BDOC for your unit or facility, you should contact the health information department.

Example of fall rate: Your facility has had four falls in the last month. The health information department reports that you had 900 BDOC last month. Your fall rate for the last month can be calculated this way:

Fall rate = (number of falls/BDOC) × 1,000 BDOC
= (4/900) × 1,000 = 4.44 per 1,000 BDOC
Interpretation: For every 1,000 BDOC, you can expect to have about four falls.

The *injury rate* tells you how many injuries per 100 falls.
Injury rate = (number of injuries/number of falls) × 100 falls

It is important to separate the injuries based on their severity, using the severity index described in the previous section. Depending on the intervention you are implementing, you may choose to measure both the major and minor injury rates. For example, if you were implementing hip protectors, you would want to see a decrease in the major injury rate, but, as a result, you may see an increase in the minor injury rate.

Example of injury rates: Your facility has had 80 falls in the last month. Of the 80 falls, 5 resulted in a minor injury, 3 resulted in a major injury such as a hip fracture, and the remainder resulted in no injury.

Minor injury rate = (5/80) × 100 = 6.25 per 100 falls (6.25%)
Major injury rate = (3/80) × 100 = 3.75 per 100 falls (3.75%)
Interpretation: 6.25% of the falls last month resulted in minor injuries, and 3.75% resulted in major injuries.

Other Important Measures

When aggregating fall data, look for trends such as falls related to toileting or repeat fallers. This can lead to focusing on reducing particular types of falls. To do this you may want to keep track of the following:

1. Where a fall occurred (specific unit or a place like the bathroom or hallway)
2. What the care recipient was doing, or attempting to do, at the time of the fall
3. The shift on which the fall occurred (for example, first, second, or third shift)

This information is categorical, and the easiest way to analyze it is by using a Pareto chart or bar graph. To aid aggregate review teams and target future interventions, you should keep track of factors that are related to each fall, such as communication issues, assistive devices, and environmental factors.

Analyzing the Data to Measure Progress

Once you have collected the data you will need to analyze the information. There are many ways to look at your data. Two methods are by using run charts or Pareto charts.

Run Charts

Run charts are used to track data over time. They are most often used to track data like fall rates or injury rates. It is important to clearly mark on the graph the months that the interventions were implemented. To show a difference you will want to take the average fall rate for the months prior to the interventions.

Example: The fall rates per 1,000 BDOC at a facility for the last year are shown in Figure 5-1.

In May, an education program was implemented and in June a program to reduce repeat fallers was implemented. The run chart for this is shown in Figure 5-2.

To see if the interventions are working, you will want to take the average fall rate prior to the interventions and after the interventions, as shown in Table 5-1.

FIGURE 5-1

Fall Rate per 1,000 BDOC

Month	Rate	Month	Rate
January	10.5	July	9.9
February	11	August	8.7
March	12	September	6.3
April	11.3	October	5.3
May	12.4	November	5.6
June	10	December	4.5

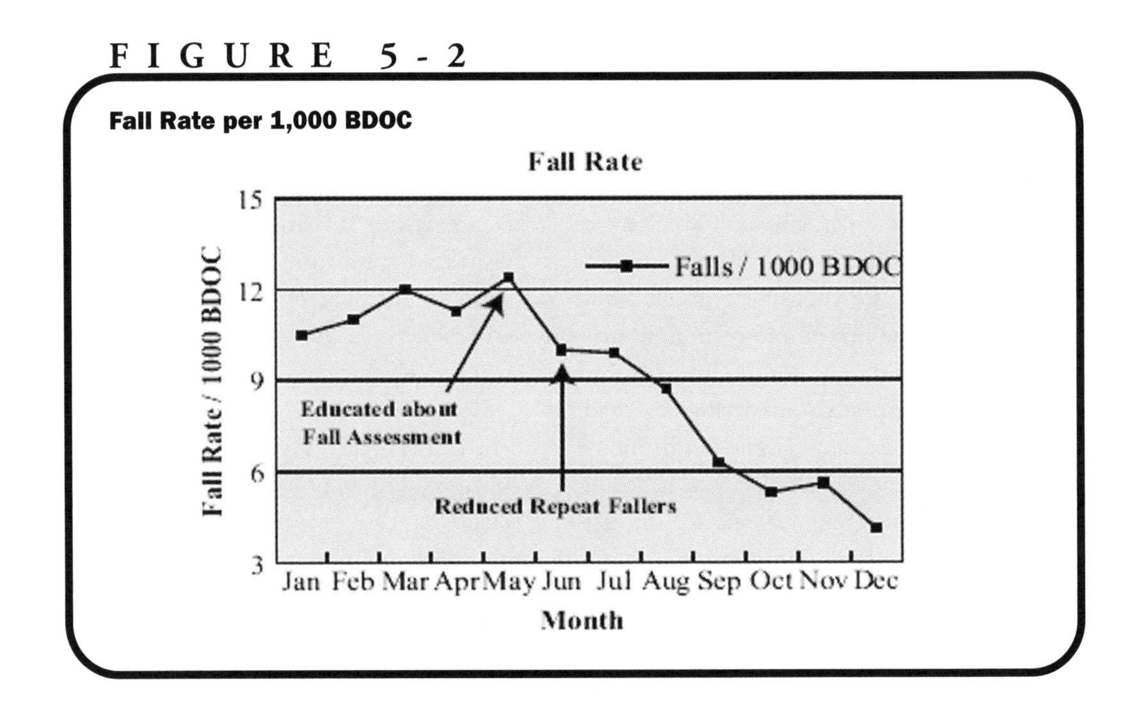

TABLE 5-1

Fall Rate Prior to Interventions and After Interventions

Month	# Falls	BDOC	Fall Rate per 1000 BDOC	Month	# Falls	BDOC	Fall Rate per 1000 BDOC
January	10	950	10.5	July	10	1010	9.9
February	11	1000	11	August	10	1150	8.7
March	15	1250	12	September	8	1275	6.3
April	13	1150	11.3	October	6	1130	5.3
May	13	1050	12.4	November	6	1080	5.6
June	11	1100	10	December	4	975	4.1
Totals	73	6500	11.2	**Totals**	44	6620	6.6

In this case, the average fall rate for January through June is as follows:

((10+11+15+13+13+11)/(950+1,000+1,250+1,150+1,050+1,100)) × 1,000 = (73/6,500) × 1,000 = 11.2 per 1,000 BDOC

The average fall rate for the months after the intervention (July–December) is as follows:

((10+10+8+6+6+4)/(1,010+1,150+1,275+1,130+1,080+975)) × 1,000 = (44/6,620) × 1,000 = 6.6 per 1,000 BDOC

This means that prior to the interventions the average fall rate was 11.2, and after the interventions the fall rate decreased to 6.6. Prior to the interventions, the facility could expect 11.2 falls per 1,000 BDOC. After the interventions, the facility could expect 6.6 falls per 1,000 BDOC.

To analyze this further you could take the variance of the data or do a statistical means test. Both of these can be done using functions in a spreadsheet program.

Bar Graphs

Bar graphs are used to visualize categorical data, such as the location of care recipient falls or what the care recipient was trying to accomplish at the time of the fall. They can be used to target interventions where there is the highest risk. For instance, if most of the falls are occurring while the care recipient is toileting, then initiating toileting schedules for at-risk care recipients may be an option. The bar graph is sorted with the largest category first and the smallest category last. It may be helpful to separate the data into separate charts, such as falls by location or shift.

Example: A facility tracked what the care recipients were attempting to do at the time of a fall. They found that the falls broke down into the categories shown in Table 5-2 on page 122.

The data graphed into the bar graph shown in Figure 5-3 on page 122.

Bar graphs can also be used to show the incidence of certain factors before and after an intervention. For instance, after implementing a frequent toileting schedule for incontinent care recipients with urgency, they found that the incidence of falls was as shown in Figure 5-4.

As the graph shows, there appears to be a difference before and after the toileting schedule was implemented.

Risk Adjustments

Comparing fall rates among different institutions can be difficult. From organization to organization, there are varying fall definitions and methods to report data. There are differ-

TABLE 5-2

Categories of Falls

Category	Number
Toileting	28
Transferring	25
Walking to bathroom	20
Transferring from chair	14
Walking in hallway	9
Rolled out of bed	5

FIGURE 5-3

Factors Related to Falls

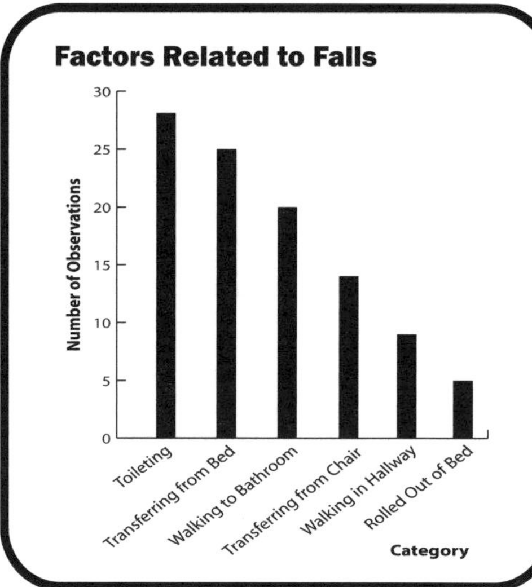

FIGURE 5-4

Patient Falls Before and After Testing

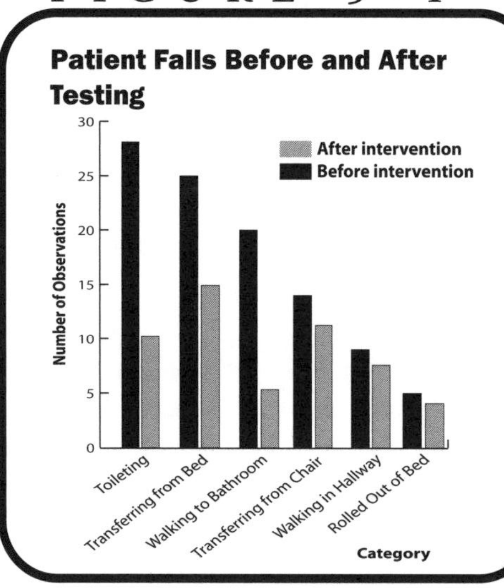

ences in settings, care recipient populations, and risk adjustments.

For example, studies reported by Janice Morse provide a range of fall rates (per 1,000 bed days) from 2.2 to 7 in acute care hospitals, 11.0 to 24.9 in long term care hospitals, and 8.0 to 19.8 in rehabilitation hospitals.[1] Elsewhere, the range of injury rates in percentages has been reported to be from 29 to 48, with 4% to 7.5% resulting in serious injuries. Some other studies have suggested that the average rate for acute care hospitals is in the range of 2.5 to 3.5 falls per care recipient for every 1,000 bed days. In reviewing such studies, it is critical to note the method and whether the data are risk-adjusted. It is important that a facility risk-adjust its data using similar definitions before making a comparison to other external organizations with "similar" populations.

For many organizations, the most useful and reliable approach to measurement is through examining its own quality indicator data over time.

Trending

Although it has been deemed valuable to trend reported care recipient falls per 1,000 care recipient days, organizations should be careful when comparing care recipient care from unit to unit, or even individual units to the overall organizational rate—much less other organizations—unless rates are risk-adjusted.

Some organizations might find more value in generating control charts for each of the units so that, over time, each unit can determine whether its processes are stable. If they are not, the data should trigger an investigation to identify possible causes and remedial actions. Regardless of whether processes are stable within a unit, areas that have relatively high reported fall rates should still look for ways to reduce their median fall rate. This process must consider the nature of the care recipient population and other factors, so that the chosen strategies are appropriate. This approach supports the use of unit trends over time, related to the implementation of strategies, and determination of whether selected strategies are effective.

Monitoring Systems

Monitoring systems of fall rates are usually established by hospitals for monthly and annual reporting purposes, according to Morse. Referring to it as a "scorecard" on the effectiveness of the program, Morse sees the fall monitoring system as an integral part of fall reduction. Used in four ways, the monitoring system does the following:

1. Enables assessment of the severity of the problem and the cost of care recipient falls. The severity statements should be used not only when planning a program, but also on a regular basis to make a case for a continuing problem.

2. Enables evaluation of the efficacy of the program institutionwide and allows for estimates of cost savings. When compared with baseline preprogram statistics, annual rates should give ongoing information about the success of the fall reduction program. However, the interpretation of these statistics should be viewed in context of staff levels, care recipient acuity data, and the fall reporting rates. At the commencement of a fall program, falls may suddenly increase because of changes in reporting rates. Fall injury rates may be a better predictor of the success of the program.

3. Assists with the identification of "hot spots" or patterns of fall incidents. These may be achieved in a number of ways, including the following:

   a. By care recipient typology—Analysis of statistics by care recipient characteristics, separate from care recipient care unit, will provide important information on patterns about who is falling. For example, statistics should be inspected against the Morse Fall Scale and by item. Do most care recipients who fall have scores that indicates they are "using the furniture" to ambulate? Why are these care recipients not provided with assistance or a walking aid?

   b. By unit or service—If most of the falls are occurring in specific units or services, special attention must be given to the causes of these falls. For example, should more staffing be provided? Should an environmental scan be conducted to consider the addition of more handrails?

   c. By "geographical" location—The locations of falls are classically bathrooms or at the bedside. Other hot spots must also be considered (for example, a foyer or doorway). Safety begins with awareness of the problem—use your monitoring system to its full capacity.

   d. By particular equipment—Falls may be repeatedly occurring from wheelchairs or involving walkers—look for such patterns.

   e. By circumstance (including time of fall)—What are care recipients doing when they fall? Transferring? Rushing to the bathroom? Consider care recipient activities in your institutionwide monitoring system so that staff may be altered to address these patterns.

4. Enables immediate responsiveness to multiple (repeated) falls. The monitoring system may provide instant feedback to staff about type, location, and care recipient activity of a fall. Because the second and subsequent fall may occur when the care recipient is doing the same thing, this information can be incorporated into the care recipient's care plan, and a repeated fall may be circumvented.

Comparing Data to Reduce Falls and Measure Results

Inhibited motor skills, poor vision, multiple medications—the list of risk factors related to falls in care recipients has been discussed in detail in this book. Organizations may already be collecting data on falls as part of the minimum data set (MDS) requirements, but they may not be getting as much use from these data as they could. Comparing results from a variety of MDS measures can not only help an organization analyze relationships among different areas, but assist an organization in the evaluation of a fall reduction program and point an organization in the right direction in reducing future falls.

The information gathered must be interpreted for the population served. For example, an organization must collect data on the number of falls that occur and then interpret the significance for the organization. The federal definition of a fall encompasses any situation in which the resident touches the floor—even if he or she felt dizzy and simply sat down or was assisted to the floor. This definition of a fall can encumber the analysis of the root causes of injuries associated with a fall. With the increasing emphasis on proactive care recipient safety efforts, the organization needs all the information it can get to pinpoint trouble spots, evaluate performance, and focus attention to eliminate those hazards.

When a surveyor visits an organization, he or she wants to know that the organization and staff have information, that they have used it, that they are aggregating their data, that the numbers are meaningful, and that they have enough data trended so that they can start to make some conclusions. For example, an organization that does not have a formal human resources department may not think of comparing staffing data (how many staff were on a unit; how many were full-time, part-time, or contracted) with fall data. However, this information would be available through whatever company or department handles the facility's payroll services.

Falls usually occur in conjunction with several possible factors. By looking at data for different measures together, an organization can build a picture of what is actually taking place in its facility and how it relates to the elements of its fall reduction plan. The scenario on multiple measures (page 138) demonstrates how data can be used to increase an organization's knowledge of why falls occur and where there may be room for improvement. The actual measures chosen will depend on an organization's care recipient population and the facility's specific processes and needs. These data will offer solid answers to surveyors' questions about how data are being used. They will also provide an organization with important answers to how its fall reduction program is performing.[4]

You are ready to start analyzing data on several measures that you think are related to falls. What do you do? First, you need to monitor the falls themselves and separate your data on the basis of specific characteristics. For example, you may decide to look at total number of falls, falls with minor injuries, falls with serious injuries, and observed (as opposed to unobserved) falls. Before you begin, make sure you have defined each of these measures—what constitutes a minor or a major injury, and so on—and of course define "falls." You can enter your results in a matrix, which might look like the one in Table 5-3.

You may find it helpful to create a multiple-line graph like the one in Figure 5-5 so that you have a picture of how the results compare. If you are dealing with more than one type of care recipient population—say, one that is alert but has limited mobility and an Alzheimer's unit

TABLE 5-3

Types of Falls per 100 Resident Days

Time Period	12/00	3/01	6/01	9/01	12/01	3/02	6/02	9/02	12/02
Total number of falls	6	5	12	4	5	3	9	5	6
Falls with minor injuries	3	1	6	1	0	2	4	1	2
Falls with serious injuries	0	2	4	1	0	0	3	0	1
Observed falls	2	1	1	3	4	3	1	3	2

FIGURE 5-5

Multiline Graph Results

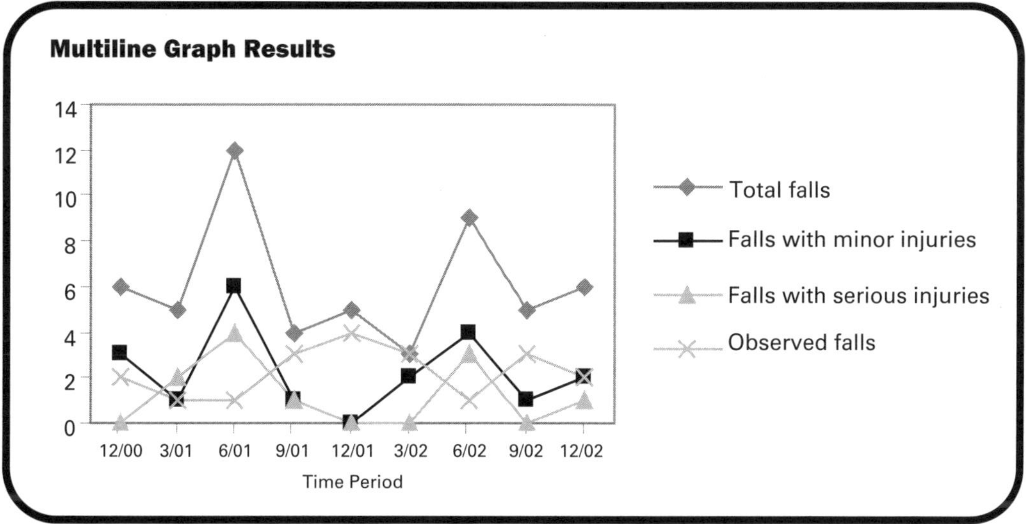

where care recipients are fairly healthy—it will probably help you to break out results by population as well. From the matrix and the graph shown here, you can see that there seems to be an inverse relationship between how many falls resulted in serious injury and how many were observed.

When you have stratified your fall data, think about other measures that might be related to the results you already have. For example, if a lack of observation is associated with an increase in serious injuries, you may want to look at staffing data (how many full-time and part-time staff were on the unit) and on what shift the falls occurred (in the middle of the night, during meals, and so forth). It may also help to use care recipient characteristics, such as multiple medications, that are associated with an increased risk of falls. You can obtain staff data from your human resources department or your payroll records, and care recipient characteristics through a chart or incident record review. This step might yield a matrix and graph that look like the ones in Table 5-4 and Figure 5-6.

Based on a comparison of these results, you may conclude that low staffing numbers—perhaps due to insufficient coverage during vacations or to coverage by contract staff who were unfamiliar with care recipients' needs—contributed greatly to the number of injuries sustained from falls. Thus, staffing issues would be a top priority in your improvement plans.

However, in this example the data also show

TABLE 5-4

Number of Falls and Risk Factors per 100 Resident Days

Time Period	12/00	3/01	6/01	9/01	12/01	3/02	6/02	9/02	12/02
Falls with injuries (serious and minor)	3	3	10	2	0	2	7	1	3
Number of full-time staff per shift	4	4	3	4	5	4	3	4	4
More than 9 medications	2	2	3	0	0	0	2	1	0
Use of glasses/hearing aid	2	3	8	2	0	1	5	1	1

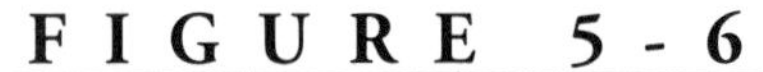

FIGURE 5-6

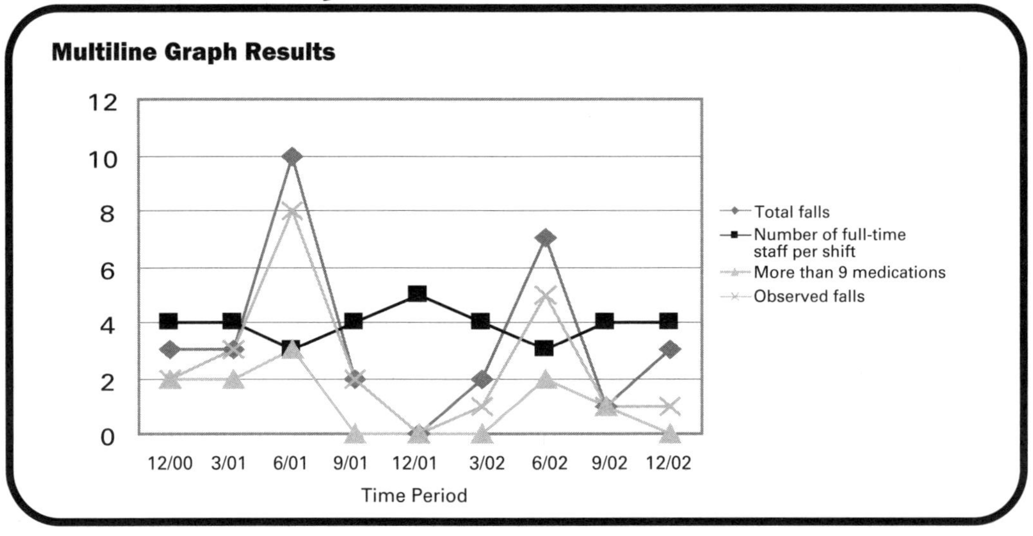

that a majority of the care recipients who were injured had impaired vision or hearing. This might be a staffing issue in that there may be no one to remind care recipients to put on their glasses or hearing aids. It also suggests that you may want to reassess the physical environment for anything that presents a challenge for care recipients who cannot see or hear well.

Performance Data Standards for Improvement

As the previous example illustrates, performance improvement is an ongoing process that involves measuring the functioning of important processes and services and, when indicated, identifying changes that enhance performance. These changes are incorporated into new or existing work processes, products, or services, and performance is monitored to ensure that the improvements are sustained.

According to the Joint Commission's standards manuals, performance improvement activities are based on outcomes of care, treatment, and services. Leaders establish a planned, systematic, and organizationwide approach(es) to performance improvement. They set priorities for performance improvement and ensure that the disciplines representing the scope of care, treatment, and services across the organization work collaboratively to plan and implement improvement activities.

An important aspect of improving organization performance is effectively reducing factors that contribute to unanticipated adverse events and/or outcomes. Unanticipated adverse events and/or outcomes may be caused by poorly designed systems, system failures, or errors. Reducing unanticipated adverse events and/or unanticipated outcomes requires an environment in which care recipients, their families, and organization staff and leaders can identify and manage actual and potential risks to safety. Such an environment encourages the following:

- Recognizing and acknowledging risks and unanticipated adverse events
- Initiating actions to reduce these risks and unanticipated adverse events
- Reporting internally on risk reduction initiatives and their effectiveness
- Focusing on processes and systems
- Minimizing individual blame or retribution for involvement in an unanticipated adverse event
- Investigating factors that contribute to unanticipated adverse events, and sharing that acquired knowledge both internally and with other organizations

The leaders are responsible for fostering such an environment both through personal example and by supporting effective responses to actual occurrences of unanticipated adverse events; ongoing proactive reduction of safety risks to residents; and integration of safety priorities into the design and redesign of all relevant organization processes, functions, and services. Sidebar 5-1, below, describes the Joint Commission standards that apply to this system of monitoring, measuring, and responding. For more on assessing and scoring your performance compliance, see the Joint Commission's standards manuals.

SIDEBAR 5-1

Joint Commission Improving Organization Performance (PI) Standards

Standard PI.1.10

The organization collects data to monitor its performance.

Rationale for PI.1.10

Data help determine performance improvement priorities. The data collected for high-priority and required areas are used to monitor the stability of existing processes, identify opportunities for improvement, identify changes that lead to improvement, or sustain improvement. Data collection helps identify specific areas that require further study. These areas are determined by considering the information provided by the data about process stability, risks, sentinel events, and priorities set by the leaders. Data may come from internal sources such as staff or external sources such as patients, referral sources, and so on. In addition, the organization identifies those areas needing improvement and identifies desired changes. Performance measures are used to determine whether the changes result in desired outcomes. The organization identifies the frequency and detail of data collection.

(continued)

SIDEBAR 5-1 (continued)

Note 1: *The organization also collects data on the evaluation and improvement of conditions in the environment and staffing effectiveness, to be discussed later.*

Note 2: *For long term care organizations that serve residents with dementia, the organization may measure performance in the following areas: psychotropic drugs, incidents, acute behavioral events, family involvement, do-not-resuscitate orders, appropriate use of services, transfers, programs that meet care recipient needs, infection control, environmental adaptations, and safety.*

Elements of Performance for PI.1.10

1. The organization collects data for priorities identified by leaders.
2. The organization considers collecting data in the following areas:
   - Staff opinions and needs
   - Staff perceptions of risks to individuals and suggestions for improving care recipient safety
   - Staff willingness to report unanticipated adverse events
3. The organization collects data on the perceptions of care, treatment, and services of care recipients, including the following:
   - Their specific needs and expectations
   - How well the organization meets these needs and expectations
   - How the organization can improve care recipient safety
   - The effectiveness of pain management, when applicable

The organization collects data that measure the performance of each of the following potentially high-risk processes, when provided:

4. Medication management
5. Blood and blood product use
6. Restraint use
7. Not applicable
8. Behavior management and treatment

9–12. Not applicable

Relevant information developed from the following activities is integrated into performance improvement initiatives. This occurs in a way consistent with any organization policies or procedures intended to preserve any confidentiality or privilege of information established by applicable law, which includes the following:

13. Risk management
14. Utilization management
15. Quality control
16. Infection control surveillance and reporting
17. Research, as applicable

(continued)

SIDEBAR 5-1 (continued)

Standard PI.2.10
Data are systematically aggregated and analyzed.

Rationale for PI.2.10
Aggregating and analyzing data means transforming data into information. Aggregating data at points in time enables the organization to judge a particular process's stability or a particular outcome's predictability in relation to performance expectations. Accumulated data are analyzed in such a way that current performance levels, patterns, or trends can be identified.

Elements of Performance for PI.2.10
1. Collected data are aggregated and analyzed.
2. Data are aggregated at the frequency appropriate to the activity or process being studied.
3. Statistical tools and techniques are used to analyze and display data.
4. Data are analyzed and compared internally over time and externally with other sources of information, when available.
5. Comparative data are used to determine if there are excessive variability or unacceptable levels of performance, when available.

Standard PI.2.20
Undesirable patterns or trends in performance are analyzed.

Elements of Performance for PI.2.20
1. Analysis is performed when data comparisons indicate that levels of performance, patterns, or trends vary substantially from those expected.
2. Analysis occurs for those topics chosen by leaders as performance improvement priorities.
3. Analysis is performed when undesirable variation occurs that changes priorities.

An analysis is performed for the following:
4. All confirmed transfusion reactions, if applicable to the organization
5. All serious adverse drug events, if applicable and as defined by the organization
6. All significant medication errors, if applicable and as defined by the organization
7. Not applicable
8. Not applicable
9. Hazardous conditions
10. Staffing effectiveness issues

Standard PI.2.30
Processes for identifying and managing sentinel events are defined and implemented.

Rationale for PI.2.30
Identifying, reporting, analyzing, and managing sentinel events can help the organization to prevent such incidents. Leaders define and implement such a program as part of the process to measure, assess, and improve the organization's performance.

(continued)

SIDEBAR 5-1 (continued)

Elements of Performance or PI.2.30

Processes for identifying and managing sentinel events include the following:

1. Defining sentinel event and communicating this definition throughout the organization. (At a minimum, the organization's definition includes those events subject to review under the Joint Commission's Sentinel Event Policy as published in its standards manuals and may include any process variation that does not affect the outcome or result in an adverse event, but for which a recurrence carries significant chance of a serious adverse outcome or result in an adverse event, often referred to as a "near miss.")
2. Reporting sentinel events through established channels in the organization and, as appropriate, to external agencies in accordance with law and regulation
3. Conducting thorough and credible root cause analyses that focus on process and system factors
4. Creating, documenting, and implementing a risk-reduction strategy and action plan that includes measuring the effectiveness of process and system improvements to reduce risk
5. The processes are implemented.

Standard PI.3.10

Information from data analysis is used to make changes that improve performance and care recipient safety and reduce the risk of sentinel events.

Elements of Performance for PI.3.10

1. The organization uses the information from data analysis to identify and implement changes that will improve the quality of care, treatment, and services.
2. The organization identifies and implements changes that will reduce the risk of sentinel events.
3. The organization uses the information from data analysis to identify changes that will improve care recipient safety.
4. Changes made to improve processes or outcomes are evaluated to ensure that they achieve the expected results.
5. Appropriate actions are undertaken when planned improvements are not achieved or sustained.

Standard PI.3.20

An ongoing proactive program for identifying and reducing unanticipated adverse events and safety risks to care recipients is defined and implemented.

Rationale for PI.3.20

Organizations should proactively seek to identify and reduce risks to the safety of care recipients. Such initiatives have the obvious advantage of preventing adverse events rather than simply reacting when they occur. This approach also avoids the barriers to understanding created by hindsight bias and the fear of disclosure, embarrassment, blame, and punishment that can happen after an event.

(continued)

SIDEBAR 5-1 (continued)

Elements of Performance for PI.3.20

The following proactive activities to reduce risks to care recipients are conducted:

1. Selecting a high-risk process to be analyzed (at least one high-risk process is chosen annually-the choice should be based in part on information published periodically by the Joint Commission about the most frequent sentinel events and risks). (A high-risk process is a process that, if not planned and/or implemented correctly, has a significant potential for impacting the safety of the care recipient.)
2. Describing the chosen process (for example, through the use of a flowchart)
3. Identifying the ways in which the process could break down or fail to perform its desired function. (The ways in which processes could break down or fail to perform its desired function are many times referred to as "the failure modes.")
4. Identifying the possible effects that a breakdown or failure of the process could have on care recipients and the seriousness of the possible effects
5. Prioritizing the potential process breakdowns or failures
6. Determining why the prioritized breakdowns or failures could occur, which may include performing a hypothetical root cause analysis
7. Redesigning the process and/or underlying systems to minimize the risk of the effects on care recipients
8. Testing and implementing the redesigned process
9. Monitoring the effectiveness of the redesigned process

The Joint Commission Staffing Effectiveness Standard

Measuring the success of an effective fall reduction program involves measuring the full spectrum of staffing effectiveness. As mentioned previously, effective staffing has been linked to positive patient/resident outcomes and improved quality and safety of care. The Joint Commission's standard for hospital, long term care, and assisted living programs (HR.1.30; HR.2.1 for assisted living) is designed to help health care organizations determine and continuously improve the effectiveness of their staffing through an objective evidence-based approach.

Staffing effectiveness is defined as the number, competency, and skill mix of staff related to the provision of needed services. According to this standard, the described goal relies on the use of relevant clinical outcome and human resources screening indicators to monitor and identify staff-related improvement opportunities in the provision of patient/resident care. In its simplest conception, this standard reflects the application of continuous quality improvement methods to the performance of staffing effectiveness.

This staffing standard requires health care organizations to collect data on relevant human resources and clinical screening indicators for a minimum of two units/divisions (populations/settings for long term care and assisted living), determine the desired performance for each indicator, trend the data over time, and analyze variation from desired performance.

Unit/division refers to the level in which staffing is planned and is provided within the organization. For example, staffing may be planned for individual units or for a group of units, such as all medical/surgical units.

Populations/settings refers to the level in which staffing is planned and is provided within the organization. For example, staffing may be provided for individual populations or settings, or may be planned for group settings or populations.

It may be appropriate to rotate the units/ divisions (populations/settings for long term care and assisted living) being monitored over time, after sufficient data have been reviewed to conclude that care on these units is stable. The use of multiple indicators increases the likelihood that existing problems will be identified and appropriately characterized. The use of nursing-sensitive measures makes it likely that problems identified will be staffing related. However, this will not be universally true—the types of root causes may be identified and will need to be addressed.

Many organizations will find that they are already collecting the types of data contemplated by this standard. Methods of data collection and tools for data analysis do not need to be sophisticated, and analysis may vary based on the availability of resources. Simple control charts or other graphics to display data may be sufficient.

The purpose of collecting data for these indicators is to screen for possible nurse staffing issues and then to analyze the underlying cause(s) when the data do not meet performance expectations. Identification of statistical correlations among measure results is not required; however, identified relationships among results may provide clues to the underlying cause(s).

The data for each screening indicator are analyzed to identify any variations from desired performance by individual measure. Variations in performance trigger further analysis to determine the cause(s) of the variation and whether staffing effectiveness issues might be affecting outcomes of care. When variation from desired performance is identified in one indicator, other indicator results are reviewed to identify information that may assist in elucidating the potential cause(s) of variation.

In the analysis of data that vary from expectations, the organization should drill down to determine the cause(s) of variation and undertake steps leading to appropriate actions that are likely to remedy identified problems. For example, analysis of the data may indicate the need for evaluation of the organization's staffing practices. If so, the organization should take specific actions to improve its performance. Examples of strategies that may be used to address identified staffing issues include the following:

- Staff recruitment
- Education/training
- Service curtailment
- Increased technology support
- Reorganization of work flow
- Provision of additional ancillary or support staff
- Adjustment of skill mix

Standard HR.1.30 is discussed in Sidebar 5-2, beginning on page 133.

The case study on page 138 serves as a real-life example of the role data play in an effective fall reduction program.

Drawing Conclusions on Fall Reduction Programs

The primary goal in measuring the effectiveness of a fall reduction program is to arrive at a base of knowledge that allows an organization to proactively respond to the conclusions of its measurements. That may involve developing strategies that sustain the strength of a program or improve particular aspects of a program.

Figures 5-7 through 5-9, beginning on page 141, contain a summary of recent studies of fall

SIDEBAR 5-2

Management of Human Resources Standard (HR) and Screening Indicators

Standard HR.1.30

The organization uses data from clinical/service screening indicators in combination with human resources screening indicators to assess and continuously improve staffing effectiveness.

Rationale for HR.1.30

Significant changes in nurse staffing level and the skill mix of nursing personnel in health care organizations raise questions about potential adverse effects on the quality and safety of patient care related to staffing effectiveness. The Joint Commission has developed a comprehensive approach to the management of staffing effectiveness that looks at staffing as more than just "numbers." The approach relies on data driven quality improvement principles and is objective and methodologically sound. Since the causes and consequences of diminished staffing effectiveness differ from organization to organization, the approach allows flexibility to reflect characteristics unique to individual health care settings.

Elements of Performance for HR.1.30

1. The organization identifies no fewer than two inpatient populations/settings for which data on staffing effectiveness are to be collected.

Note: *If the organization has only* population/setting, *the organization may collect data for that single population/setting.*

2. The organization identifies the populations/settings (no less than two) based on assessment of relevant information or risk, including the following:
   - Knowledge about staffing issues likely to impact resident safety or quality of care
   - Resident population served
   - Type of setting
   - Review of existing data (for example, incident logs, sentinel event data, performance improvement reports)
   - Input from clinical staff who provide resident care

Note: *If the organization has only one population/setting, the organization need not apply these criteria.*

3. A minimum set of four indicators are selected for each of the identified inpatient populations/settings.

Note: *Organizations are free to choose the same set, the same set in part or completely different measure sets for each identified population/setting.*

4. The organization determines the indicators for each population/setting based on assessment of relevant information or risk, including the following:
   - Knowledge about staffing issues likely to impact resident safety or quality of care
   - Resident population served
   - Type of setting
   - Review of existing data (for example, incident logs, sentinel event data, performance improvement reports)
   - Input from clinical staff who provide resident care

(continued)

SIDEBAR 5-2 (continued)

5. Of the four indicators required for each population/setting, two must be clinical/service indicators and two must be human resource indicators.
6. One of the human resource indicators and one of the clinical/service indicators must be selected from the Joint Commission's list of approved indicators*.

Note: *Additional indicators may be selected from among the organization's own indicators.*

7. All nursing staff (including registered nurses, licensed practical nurses, and nursing assistants or aides) are included in the human resource indicators for all identified populations/settings.

Note: *Decisions regarding stratification of data by discipline are left to the organization.*

8. When the organization chooses to include other practitioner groups (in addition to nursing staff) in the human resource indicators for the identified populations/settings, this decision is based on the impact the absence of such care/service providers would be expected to have on resident outcomes.
9. The organization does the following:
   - Defines the numerator and denominator for indicators chosen
   - Standardizes the data element definitions for each indicator, including those indicators applied in more than one setting
   - Determines acceptable ranges/parameters/trigger levels† for the indicators
10. The organization does the following:
    - Collects data for all indicators selected
    - Analyzes data for all indicators selected
    - Reviews all indicator data together when analyzing variation from desired performance for additional information that may assist in identifying any potential causes of variation
    - Investigates to identify any staffing effectiveness issues when indicator data varies from expected
    - Takes appropriate action in response to analyzed data
11. The organization reports at least annually to the leaders on the results of data analyses related to staffing effectiveness (see PI.1.10 and PI.2.20) and any actions taken to resolve identified problems.

List of Joint Commission Screening Indicators for Hospitals

1. Patient/family complaints/satisfaction (Clinical/Service)
2. Adverse drug events (Clinical/Service)
3. Injuries to patients (Clinical/Service)
4. Skin breakdown (Clinical/Service)
5. Pneumonia (Clinical/Service)
6. Postoperative infections (Clinical/Service)

* The Joint Commission's list of approved screening indicators consists of National Quality Forum [NQF]-endorsed voluntary consensus standards for nursing home care and Joint Commission consensus measures.

† Acceptable ranges/parameters/trigger levels may be reflective of past performance, expert opinion, expert literature, or a combination of these. The ranges/parameters/trigger levels should be reasonable goals that are possible to attain. When desired ranges/parameters/trigger levels are not met, an investigation into the cause(s) is needed.

(continued)

SIDEBAR 5-2 (continued)

7. Urinary tract infections (Clinical/Service)
8. Upper gastrointestinal bleeding (Clinical/Service)
9. Shock/cardiac arrest (Clinical/Service)
10. Length of stay (Clinical/Service)
11. Death among surgical inpatients with treatable serious complications (failure to rescue) (Clinical/Service) (National Quality Forum measure)
12. Pressure ulcer prevalence (Clinical/Service) (National Quality Forum measure)
13. Falls prevalence (Clinical/Service) (National Quality Forum measure)
14. Falls with injury (Clinical/Service) (National Quality Forum measure)
15. Restraint prevalence (vest and limb only) (Clinical/Service) (National Quality Forum measure)
16. Urinary catheter-associated urinary tract infection for intensive care unit patients (Clinical/Service) (National Quality Forum measure)
17. Central line catheter-associated blood stream infection rate for intensive care unit and high-risk nursery patients (Clinical/Service) (National Quality Forum measure)
18. Ventilator-associated pneumonia for intensive care unit and high-risk nursery patients (Clinical/Service) (National Quality Forum measure)
19. Smoking cessation counseling for acute myocardial infarction (Clinical/Service) (National Quality Forum measure)
20. Smoking cessation counseling for heart failure (Clinical/Service) (National Quality Forum measure)
21. Smoking cessation counseling for pneumonia (Clinical/Service) (National Quality Forum measure)
    a. Overtime (Human Resource)
    b. Staff vacancy rate (Human Resource)
    c. Staff satisfaction (Human Resource)
    d. Staff turnover rate (Human Resource)
    e. Understaffing as compared to organization's staffing plan (Human Resource)
    f. Staff injuries on the job (Human Resource)
    g. On-call or per diem use (Human Resource)
    h. Sick time (Human Resource)
    i. Agency staff use (Human Resource)
    j. Skill mix (registered nurse, licensed vocational nurse/licensed practical nurse, unlicensed assistive personnel, and contract) (Human Resource) (National Quality Forum measure)
    k. Nursing care hours per patient day (registered nurse, licensed practical nurse, and unlicensed assistive personnel) (Human Resource) (National Quality Forum measure)
    l. Practice Environment Scale-Nursing Work Index (PES-NWI) composite and five subscales (Human Resource) (National Quality Forum measure)
    m. Voluntary turnover (Human Resource) (National Quality Forum measure)

Note: Information on National Quality Forums National Voluntary Consensus Standards for Nursing-Sensitive Care, including the specific definitions for each indicator, can be found at http://www.qualityforum.org and at http://www.qualityforum.org/txNCappCspec2-7-04.pdf.

(continued)

SIDEBAR 5-2 (continued)

List of Joint Commission Screening Indicators for Long Term Care

1. Prevalence of pressure ulcers (Clinical/Service)
2. Resident satisfaction (Clinical/Service)
3. Family satisfaction (Clinical/Service)
4. Prevalence of falls (Clinical/Service)
5. Resident complaints (Clinical/Service)
6. Injuries to residents (Clinical/Service)
7. Family complaints (Clinical/Service)
8. Restraint use (Clinical/Service)
9. Prevalence of unintended weight loss (Clinical/Service)
10. Elopements/wandering of residents (Clinical/Service)
11. Adverse drug events (Clinical/Service)
12. Prevalence of dehydration (Clinical/Service)
13. Pain assessment and management (that is, wait time to receive medications) (Clinical/Service)
14. Urinary tract infection rate (Clinical/Service)
15. Change in resident functioning (Clinical/Service)
16. Prevalence of malnutrition (Clinical/Service)
17. Activities of daily living (ADLs) met or unmet (Clinical/Service)
18. Prevalence of urinary catheter use (Clinical/Service)
19. Average time in activities (Clinical/Service)
20. Antibiotic use (Clinical/Service)
21. Unexpected hospital admissions or emergency department visits (Clinical/Service)
22. Prevalence of untreated depression (Clinical/Service)
23. Prevalence of more than eight prescribed medications (Clinical/Service)
24. Pneumonia rate (Clinical/Service)
25. Unnecessary antipsychotic medication usage (Clinical/Service)

Chronic Care Measures

26. Residents whose need for more help with daily activities has increased (Clinical/Service) (National Quality Forum Measure)
27. Residents who lost too much weight (Clinical/Service) (National Quality Forum Measure)
28. Residents who experience moderate to severe pain during the seven-day assessment period (Clinical/Service) (National Quality Forum Measure)
29. Residents who were physically restrained during the seven-day assessment period (Clinical/Service) (National Quality Forum Measure)
30. Residents who spent most of their time in bed or in a chair in their room during the seven-day assessment period (Clinical/Service) (National Quality Forum Measure)
31. Residents with a decline in their ability to move about in their room or the adjacent corridor (Clinical/Service) (National Quality Forum Measure)
32. Residents with a urinary tract infection (Clinical/Service) (National Quality Forum Measure)
33. Residents with worsening of a depressed or anxious mood (Clinical/Service) (National Quality Forum Measure)

(continued)

SIDEBAR 5-2 (continued)

Chronic Care Measure Pairs

34. High-risk residents with pressure ulcers AND average-risk residents with pressure ulcers (Clinical/Service) (National Quality Forum Measure)
35. Residents who frequently lose control of the bowel or bladder (low-risk) AND residents who have a catheter in the bladder at any time during the 14-day assessment period (Clinical/Service) (National Quality Forum Measure)

Post-Acute Care Measures

36. Recently hospitalized residents with symptoms of delirium (Clinical/Service) (National Quality Forum Measure)
37. Recently hospitalized residents who experienced moderate to severe pain at any time during the seven-day assessment period (Clinical/Service) (National Quality Forum Measure)
38. Recently hospitalized residents with pressure ulcers (Clinical/Service) (National Quality Forum Measure)

Measures for All Nursing Home Residents

39. Pneumococcal polysaccharide vaccination of residents age 65 or older (Clinical/Service) (National Quality Forum Measure)
40. Influenza vaccination for all nursing home residents (Clinical/Service) (National Quality Forum Measure)
41. Staff vacancy rate (Human Resource)
42. Staff turnover rate (Human Resource)
43. Staff satisfaction (Human Resource)
44. Use of overtime (Human Resource)
45. Staff injury rate (Human Resource)
46. Nursing hours per resident day (registered nurse, licensed practical nurse, certified nursing assistant) compared to baseline such as actual versus planned or budgeted (Human Resource)
47. Staff training hours (Human Resource)
48. Agency usage/contract staff (Human Resource)
49. Understaffing as compared to organization's staffing plan (Human Resource)
50. Use of sick time (Human Resource)
51. Activity staff hours per resident day (Human Resource)
52. Number of dietary staff hours per resident day (Human Resource)
53. Number of housekeeping staff hours per resident day (Human Resource)
54. Average response time for consultation order (Human Resource)
55. Nurse staffing hours (Human Resource) (National Quality Forum Measure)

Note: Additional information on nursing home care measures can be found at http://www.qualityforum.org.

EXAMPLE 5-1

Veterans Administration Pilots Organizations Using Good Data Measures to Reduce Fall Injuries

Falls are the number one cause of reported adverse events in Veterans Administration (VA) facilities. Of the 620 serious falls reported to the VA Adverse Events Registry in 1999, 60% resulted in hip fractures and 7% resulted in death. Given that, a collaborative of 37 teams from VA hospitals and nursing homes set out to reduce falls and injuries due to falls. During the eight-month effort, teams tracked monthly fall and injury rates as they implemented a variety of interventions. The overall fall rate decreased slightly, from 6.84 falls per 1,000 bed days of care (BDOC) to 6.42. However, the overall major injury rate dropped 62%.

"The major injuries were our real focus because the goal is to keep patients from getting hurt, not just from falling," says Peter Mills, Ph.D., M.S., associate director, Field Office, VA National Center for Patient Safety (NCPS), White River Junction, Vermont, who directed the collaborative.

Universal Measures

Essential to the project was use of universal measures across the collaborative, as well as measures specific to each organization, depending on the intervention being implemented. For starters, many of the facilities had not been using a consistent definition of falls. The VA uses the following universal definition:

> *Loss of upright position that results in landing on the floor, the ground, or an object or furniture, or a sudden uncontrolled, unintentional, nonpurposeful, downward displacement of the body to the floor/ground or hitting another object like a chair or a stair.*

The VA definition does not specify witnessed versus unwitnessed falls, explains Julia Neily, R.N., M.S., nurse associate director at the NCPS Field Office. "But we believe that reporting may have become more inclusive with more unwitnessed falls counted," says Neily.

In addition, many organizations implemented the Morse Fall Scale to identify patients at risk for falls. After developing staff education programs, policies and guidelines, and inter-rater reliability systems to test the scale's validity, the majority of collaborative participants have now opted to use this tool.

One reason the VA Medical Center in Bath, New York, joined the collaborative was to determine an effective fall risk screen for its high-risk patient population, something its then-current screening tool was not doing. "By standardizing the way we defined falls, identified those patients at risk for falls, and collected data, we were able to have reliable, valid measures," says Karen Strobel, R.N., nurse manager.

"'How do we measure improvement?' was our emphasis from the start," says Neily. "For every fall, ask, 'Did we do everything we could do?' Measure what you are doing right instead of just

(continued)

EXAMPLE 5-1 (continued)

tracking rates," advises Neily. The most successful teams implemented several interventions, sometimes focusing attention on one type.

Medication Formulary

The highlight of the 160-bed Bath nursing home's program was a medication formulary because certain classes of medications are associated with an increased risk for falls. The work group analyzed and trended data from adverse drug reaction reports to develop the formulary and then conduct a monthly medication review. When notified of a fall, a pharmacist checked the resident's medication profile for use of any formulary drug and made recommendations to the doctor. Bath reduced falls by 57% in the 36-bed target unit.

Toileting Program

The VA Medical Center in Manchester, New Hampshire, took a more focused approach when data (from risk management, quality monitoring, and incident reports) revealed that 30% of falls were related to toileting. The work group set up a toileting program, that brought the patient to the bathroom or offered a urinal or bedpan on a schedule. High-risk patients entered in the program needed help with toileting but were likely to try it independently.

"We set up an individualized schedule and didn't just toilet the patient every two hours," says Sandra Pascuci, R.N., minimal data set coordinator at the 120-bed skilled nursing facility. A toileting worksheet monitors nursing compliance and determines the program's effectiveness. "If someone is toileted 4 times a day, seven days a week, and had results 25 out of the 28 times, then we know the scheduling program is working," she says. The program has also helped identify other related interventions. Although fall rates were not reduced, minor injury rates declined by 14%, with no major injuries.

Assistive Devices

Using protective and assistive devices was essential to the falls program at the VA Medical Center in Washington, D.C. The work group tracked when equipment contributed to falls or injuries and also did a root cause analysis, which helped check use of appropriate equipment.

"Documentation in the postfall assessment form about equipment in use during the fall helped us collect measurable data," says Chandresh Mehta, R.P.T., supervisor of physical therapy, Geriatric and Extended Care. The work group also received daily alerts of falls that included potential interventions. Repeat falls were identified for immediate interventions. Staff competency was measured through in-services and demonstrations using the devices. The average fall rate dropped from 10.69 to 8.67 per 1,000 BDOC, with no major injuries.

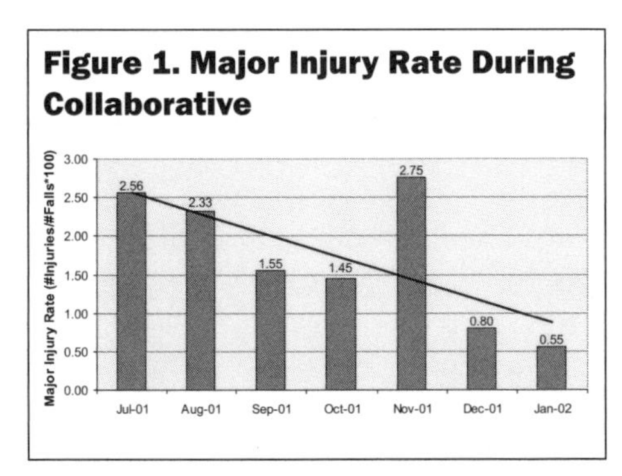

(continued)

EXAMPLE 5-1 (continued)

Safe Rooms

Similarly, the work group at the VA Medical Center in Madison, Wisconsin, chose to focus largely on the environment because an aggregated review of the fall incident reports from the previous year showed a pattern. Patients were falling by the exit side of the bed, says Bruce Kramer, R.N., B.S.N., nurse manager. The work group learned through patient and staff interviews that patients often fell because they stood up to go to the bathroom or use the urinal, or they slipped after spilling something on the floor.

Patients scoring high on the Morse Scale were assigned to a "safe room" piloted on a 22-bed general medical telemetry unit. A safe room has devices such as nonskid floor mats and a commode placed at a 90-degree angle to the bed. Trained nurses did room checks using a fall reduction checklist to determine staff competency and device effectiveness. Additionally, patients were reinterviewed about the most effective interventions. Falls were reduced by 18%, with no major injuries reported.

Sharing Data

All work groups shared data with their staff and senior leaders through presentations and their intranet, with collaborative thorough monthly reports, and also informally via their e-mail list. After the VA sites experienced success on the pilot test units, they expanded the fall program throughout their respective organizations. Many have gone on to add interventions.

Use process measures to check and test your interventions, suggests Mills. "When you start a new process, it's helpful to have simple ways to track that it is being done. It's one thing to deploy a change. It's another to see if it's changing clinician practice.[5]

reduction programs by Rein Tideiksaar, Ph.D. Tideiksaar also looks at the processes followed and the conclusions drawn from them.

As suggested by the studies above, several structural or organizational factors play a crucial role in the implementation of fall reduction programs. Some of the most important are the following:

Having an educational program aimed at increasing awareness of the problem, risk factors, and strategies. Staff should perceive that falls are a serious problem and, most important, believe that falls can be reduced.

Having a facilitywide approach to fall reduction, including a multidisciplinary committee or team with responsibility for designing, implementing, and evaluating fall reduction activities. Floor staff must play an active role in the design and implementation of the program.

Having administrative support for the program. Fall reduction programs can be successfully implemented only with strong leadership and adequate resources for the program.

FIGURE 5-7

Fall Prevention in Residential Care: A Cluster, Randomized, Controlled Trial

The purpose of this study was to establish the effectiveness of a fall prevention program in reducing falls and injurious falls in older residential care residents. Fourteen residential care homes in Auckland, New Zealand, were randomly selected for the study. Subjects included all older residents (n = 628, 95% participation rate). The intervention consisted of residential care staff, using existing resources, implemented systematic individualized fall risk management for all residents using a fall risk assessment tool, high-risk logo, and strategies to address identified risks. Outcome measurements included number of residents sustaining a fall, falls, and injurious fall incidence rates. Results showed that during 12 months of follow-up, 103 (43%) residents in the control group and 173 (56%) residents in the intervention group fell. There was a significantly higher incidence rate of falls in intervention homes than in control homes during the intervention period after adjusting for dependency level (type of home), baseline fall rate, and clustering. There was no difference in the injurious fall incidence rate or incidence of serious injuries. The researchers concluded that the fall prevention intervention did not reduce falls or injury from falls, and that low intensity intervention may be worse than usual care.

FIGURE 5-8

Effectiveness of Targeted Fall Prevention Program in Subacute Hospital Setting: Randomized, Controlled Trial

The purpose of this study was to assess the effectiveness of a targeted, multiple-intervention fall prevention program in reducing falls and injuries related to falls in three subacute wards in a metropolitan hospital specializing in rehabilitation and care of elderly patients. Subjects included 626 men and women age 38 to 99 years (average 80 years) who were recruited from consecutive admissions to subacute hospital wards. The intervention consisted of a fall risk alert card with information brochure, exercise program, education program, and hip protectors. Outcome measures included incidence rate of falls, injuries related to falls, and proportion of participants who experienced one or more falls during their stay in the hospital. Results showed that subjects in the intervention group (n = 310) experienced 30% fewer falls than participants in the control group (n = 316). This difference was significant and was most obvious after 45 days of observation. In the intervention group there was a trend for a reduction in the proportion of participants who experienced falls, and 28% fewer falls resulted in injury. The researchers concluded that a targeted multiple-intervention fall prevention program reduces the incidence of falls in the subacute hospital setting.

FIGURE 5-9

Fall Prevention Revisited: A Call for a New Approach

The purpose of this study was to test a fall prevention program in an acute medical area that was reevaluated five years later to determine if the effects were sustainable. Study design included two groups of patients admitted before and after the program. Variables such as staffing, equipment, environment, and routines were controlled. However, because of ethical approval constraints, some variables such as age, mental status, mobility, and gender were not. The program included a risk assessment tool, a choice of interventions, a graphic that alerted others to "at-risk patients," and simple patient and staff education. Data were collected using incident forms, and a formula was used to calculate a rate of falls. Results showed that the fall rate was significantly reduced. In the next five years the fall rate increased to preprogram levels. Compliance with the program had deteriorated. No definitive answers to explain noncompliance were found. It was concluded that more rigorous research into fall prevention is needed, but it may be more useful to direct research toward examining nursing work and increasing nurse autonomy in fall prevention.

EXAMPLE 5-2

Fall Prevention in Frail Elderly Nursing Home Residents: A Challenge to Case Management (Part I and Part II)

Parts I and II of this article examine the impact of a fall prevention program on the fall incidents among the residents in a nursing home. It was hypothesized that a diagnostic, therapeutic, and preventive approach should be used for nursing home residents identified as being at high risk for falls in order to reduce the number of fall incidents and to improve quality of life for this vulnerable population. The program effectively targeted both intrinsic and extrinsic factors to reduce risks facing the residents. The effectiveness of the program was evaluated by examining changes in the rate of falls after the program was implemented. The results identified that a multifaceted program, one that utilized multiple personalized interventions, was effective in reducing the fall rate of frail nursing home residents and that muscle-strengthening interventions may be beneficial for this vulnerable population. Program outcomes verified that case managers can impact quality of life for frail elderly nursing home residents by promoting their independence and safety, and postponing problems resulting from inactivity. Part I discussion includes the background and process of a fall program and factors contributing to the occurrence of falls. Part II examines the interdisciplinary team approach to assessment, method, and implementing strategies for an effective fall prevention program. Tools used for prevention, monitoring, and investigation of falls are detailed in Part II.

EXAMPLE 5-3

Reducing Falls and Fall-Related Injuries in the VA System

The purpose of this study was to describe the process, outcomes, and team success factors of a multifacility quality improvement effort designed to reduce falls and fall-related injuries among inpatients. Thirty-seven teams from VA hospitals, veterans nursing homes, and one private facility completed an eight-month facilitated quality improvement project. Participating teams tracked fall and injury rates and reported on the interventions implemented. Though the overall fall rate decreased only slightly, the overall major injury rate dropped 62%, from 2.14 major injuries per 100 falls at baseline to 0.82 major injuries per 100 falls at project completion. This represents an average reduction of 40.9 major injuries per month for the group and a direct care cost savings of between $667,569 and $765,934 per month. The following organizational factors (staff support, strong leadership, and conflict management skills) and interventions (toileting interventions, use of signage to identify high-risk patients, use of hip pads, environmental interventions, staff education, and postfall assessments) were associated with the greatest reductions in major injury rates. The researchers concluded that facilitated quality improvement efforts were successful at reducing severe fall-related injuries and was cost-effective.

Although the literature on preventing falls in hospitals and nursing homes is widely available, implementing effective fall prevention programs remains a major challenge. According to Rein Tideiksaar, Ph.D., based on evidence-based research and expert opinion, it appears that programs of multiple interventions that target patients/residents based on individualized/ongoing fall risk and postfall assessments are likely to be the most successful. But this might not be enough.

References

1. Morse, J.M.: Enhancing the safety of hospitalization by reducing patient falls. *Am J Infect Control* 30:376–80, Jun. 2002.
2. National Center for Patient Safety (NCPS): *VHA NCPS Falls Toolkit.* May 2004. http://www.va.gov/ncps/SafetyTopics/fallstoolkit/notebook/index.html (accessed Feb. 9, 2005).
3. Chang J.T., et al.: Interventions for the prevention of falls in older adults: Systematic review and meta-analysis of randomized clinical trials. *BMJ* 328:1–7, Mar. 2004.
4. Joint Commission Resources: Measuring Up. *Joint Commission Benchmark* 5:4–5, Apr. 2003.
5. Tideiksaar R.: Literature review of the month. *RN+ Newsletter* 6:1–5, Jun. 2004.

GLOSSARY

AAFP American Academy of Family Physicians.

Action planning sessions Meetings conducted by trained line managers to identify the strategies that the organization intends to implement to reduce the risk of sentinel events occurring in the future. The planning sessions should address responsibility for implementation, oversight, pilot testing as appropriate, time lines, and strategies for measuring the effectiveness of the actions.

ADE Adverse drug event. Any incident in which the use of a medication (drug or biologic) at any dose, a medical device, or a special nutritional product (for example, dietary supplement, medical food) may have resulted in an adverse outcome in a patient.

ADLs Activities of daily living.

Adverse outcomes Negative results, such as an individual experiencing a fall despite the use of a fall reduction program in the health care facility. An untoward, undesirable, and usually unanticipated event, such as death of a patient, an employee, or a visitor in a health care organization. Incidents such as patient or resident falls or improper administration of medications are also considered adverse events, even if there is no permanent effect on the patient or resident.

AHA American Hospital Association.

AHRQ Agency for Healthcare Research and Quality.

Anesthesia A drug, administered for medical or surgical purposes, that induces partial or total loss of sensation and may be topical, local, regional, or general, depending on the method of administration and area of the body affected.

Anticholinergics A substance that opposes or blocks the action of acetylcholine. May predispose individuals to fall.

Antihypertensives A drug or treatment that reduces high blood pressure. May predispose individuals to fall.

Assessment The act of assessing an individual to determine if he or she is likely to experience a fall. Health care professionals also complete an assessment of an individual who has recently fallen to determine if treatment is necessary.

Assisted living A living arrangement in which people with special needs, especially seniors with disabilities, reside in a facility that provides help with everyday tasks such as bathing, dressing, and taking medication.

Benchmarking Continuous measurement of a process, product, or service compared to those of the toughest competitor, to those considered industry leaders, or to similar activities in the organization, in order to find and implement ways to improve it.

Caregiver A person who makes decisions for a care recipient based on his or her best interests. A caregiver may also help a care recipient walk, administer medications, and act as a liaison between the individual and the health care professionals.

Care plan or plan of action A care plan provides a detailed guide for all caregivers who are involved with an individual's care.

Care recipient A person receiving care, such as a patient or a resident.

CDC Centers for Disease Control and Prevention.

Communication The exchange of thoughts, messages, or information, as by speech, signals, writing, or behavior. Communication can be verbal and nonverbal.

Competence A specific range of skill, knowledge, or ability.

Continuous quality improvement Ongoing positive changes involving the quality of care in a health care organization.

Continuum of care The process of care given to a consumer from the time he or she enters a health care facility through his or her follow-up treatment and recovery.

Control chart Illustrates whether a variation in a process is statistically in control. Helps to identify root causes and opportunities for improvement, and also helps implement and monitor improvements.

Critical access hospital A hospital in a rural setting.

Dementia Deterioration of intellectual faculties, such as memory, concentration, and judgment, resulting from an organic disease or a disorder of the brain. It is sometimes accompanied by emotional disturbance and personality changes.

Diuretic A substance or drug that tends to increase the discharge of urine. May predispose individuals to fall.

Electronic health information A care recipient's health information that is saved in an electronic file instead of on paper.

Environment of care (EC) The setting where an individual receives treatment, such as a hospital, long term care facility, ambulatory care facility, and so forth.

ESC Evidence of Standards Compliance.

Fall An unplanned descent to the floor or an unintended event resulting in a person coming to rest on the ground, floor, or other lower level not due to any intentional movement or extrinsic force such as a stroke, fainting, or seizure.

Fall reduction program A program implemented by an organization to reduce the occurrence of patient or resident falls.

Feedback Positive and negative comments indicated on safety culture assessments that lead to culture change.

HEDIS Health Plan Employer Data and Information Set.

Home care Health care provided in the individual's home.

Hospital Bed Safety Workgroup Established in April 1999 by the Food and Drug Administration in partnership with representatives from the hospital bed industry, national health care organizations, patient advocacy groups, and other federal agencies. The work group's goal is to improve the safety of beds for individuals in all health care settings who are most vulnerable to the risk of entrapment.

Hypotension Abnormally low blood pressure. Orthostatic hypotension lowers blood pressure after standing up, and postprandial hypotension lowers blood pressure after a meal.

Information management The planning, budgeting, control, and exploitation of the information resources in an organization.

Joint Commission's Sentinel Event Advisory Group A team of individuals who review sentinel event standards and compile the Sentinel Event Database.

Line graph A diagram of lines made by connected data points that represent successive changes in the value of a variable quantity or quantities.

Long term care The health and personal care services provided to chronically ill, aged, disabled, or developmentally disabled persons in an institution or in the place of residence. Services include long term care, subacute care, dementia, special care, and long term care pharmacy. These persons are not in an acute phase of illness, but require convalescent, physical supportive, and/or restorative services on a long-term basis.

Management self-assessment tools These instruments are intended to be used by multidisciplinary teams to promote a culture for sharing information, fostering teamwork, routinely assessing the risk of errors and adverse events, and involving patients or residents and families in care delivery.

Medical history A record of health problems and the treatments received for those problems for an individual's entire life.

Medication error An error involving medications, such as administering the wrong medication for a person's disease.

Medication management Managing the distribution, administration, and use of medications in a health care facility.

Medication use management The proper use of medications that are prescribed to specific individuals.

Mobility The ability to move unaided.

Multidisciplinary team A group of health care professionals from a variety of backgrounds who work together for a common goal, such as improving patient or resident safety.

National Patient Safety Goals National Patient Safety Goals and their requirements are a series of specific actions that accredited organizations are expected to take in order to prevent medical errors such as miscommunication among caregivers, unsafe use of infusion pumps, and medication mix-ups. A panel of national safety experts has determined that taking these simple proven steps will reduce devastating medical errors.

NCQA National Committee for Quality Assurance.

Nursing care Care provided to an individual by a nurse in a hospital facility.

Occupational therapy Physical therapy involving the use of crafts and hobbies for the rehabilitation of handicapped or convalescing patients, especially for emotionally disturbed individuals.

Outcome measure A culture change as a result of patient or resident safety programs and interventions. A measure that indicates the result of the performance (or nonperformance) of a function(s) or process(es).

Pareto chart A special form of vertical bar graph that displays information in such a way that priorities for process improvement can be established. It shows the relative importance of all data and is used to direct efforts to the largest improvement.

Patient A consumer who receives health care in a hospital.

Periodic Performance Review A self-assessment conducted by health care organizations to check their compliance to standards.

Pharmacist A person trained in pharmacy.

Plan-Do-Study-Act (PDSA) A four-part method for discovering and correcting assignable causes to improve the quality of processes. *Synonyms*: Deming cycle, Shewhart cycle.

Polypharmacy When five or more different drugs are prescribed concurrently.

Reassessment To assess an individual again.

Resident A consumer receiving health care in a long term care facility.

Risk factors A previous event or condition that makes a person susceptible to falling in the future. Risk factors can be intrinsic or extrinsic.

Root cause analysis A process for identifying the basic or causal factor(s) that underlie variation in performance, including the occurrence or possible occurrence of a sentinel event.

Safety culture assessment tools These tools help organizations analyze and understand their settings and prepare for making changes regarding safety. They can take a managerial or staff perspective, or combined elements of both.

Self-report surveys These assessments focus on the perceptions of the working environment from the perspective of staff members. The employees that are specifically involved in the care of patients answer the surveys instead of having an outsider observe the environment.

Sentinel event An unexpected occurrence involving death or serious physical or psychological injury, or the risk thereof. *Serious injury* specifically includes loss of limb or function. The phrase *or the risk thereof* includes any process variation for which a recurrence would carry a significant chance of a serious adverse outcome. Such events are called *sentinel* because they signal the need for immediate investigation and response.

Sentinel Event Database compiled by the Joint Commission An organized, comprehensive collection of sentinel event data.

Staffing effectiveness The ability of staff members in a health care facility to be effective in their interactions with patients and adherence to standards.

Transfer When a care recipient stops his or her care at one health care facility and moves to another facility to continue the treatment.

Transitional care unit A health care facility that provides individuals who have had an illness or injury but no longer need to be hospitalized with a place to receive continued skilled care until they are able to care for themselves or move to another appropriate care setting.

U.S. Pharmacopeia's Safe Medication Use Expert Committee A nonprofit nongovernmental organization that sets standards for identity, strength, purity, nomenclature, labeling, and packaging of drug products and related articles. This organization is cited in federal and state statutes, and its standards are enforceable by the U.S. Food and Drug Administration.

Veterans Health Administration (VHA) An organization that provides a broad spectrum of medical, surgical, and rehabilitative care to veterans and their families.

Voluntary Hospitals of America A health care provider alliance of more than 2,200 not-for-profit health care organizations. This organization provides industry-leading supply chain management services and facilitates the development of member networks to drive sustainable results.

INDEX

A

AAFP (American Academy of Family Physicians), 19
Accidental falls
  definition, 15, 67
  extrinsic risk factors, 18
  frequency of, 15
  intervention strategies, 86
Accident/incident investigation form, 111
Action planning sessions for culture improvement, 11
Acute care fall reduction program, 142
Adverse events
  blame and shame culture, 3
  medication errors, 18
  nonpunitive culture promotion, 5–6
Advisory Committee on the Safety of Nuclear Installations, 5
Agency for Healthcare Research and Quality safety culture assessment, 6
American Academy of Family Physicians (AAFP), 19
American Geriatrics Society (AGS) Panel on Falls Prevention, 101, 103–4
American Hospital Association (AHA), *Strategies for Leadership*, 5
American Medical Directors Association (AMDA) Falls and Fall Risk Clinical Practice Guidelines, 55, 83, 84
Anticipated physiologic falls
  definition, 15, 67–68
  frequency of, 15
  intervention strategies, 86
  precautionary strategies, 86
"Assessing the Risk of Falls" (Perell), 65–66
Assessment and reassessment. *See also specific types of assessment*
  elements of assessment, 63
  fall evaluations, 61
  frequency of, 88, 90–91
  importance of, 51–52
  intensity of, 70, 78
  intervention strategies, 35–38
  measuring benefits of, 78
  medication-induced falls, 25, 36–38, 41, 42, 64–65
  physical assessment after a fall, 55, 56
  postfall checklists, 55, 56, 57
  process for, 37, 83, 84
  as root cause of falls, 30, 31
  staff education and training on, 61
  team approach to, 36, 51, 52–54
  timing of, 55
Assessment and reassessment tools, 37
  categories of tools, 65–66
  choosing a tool, 66–67, 70
  fall cause analysis tool, 58, 60
  Get Up & Go Test, 61, 66
  measuring benefits of, 78
  as part of fall reduction program, 51–52
  pilot study of, 58
  score-based tool, 58, 59
  stroke patients, 70
Assisted living organizations
  assessment for medication-induced falls, 25
  fall risk reduction (National Patient Safety Goal 9), 2
  residential care fall reduction program, 141
  staffing effectiveness standard, 131
Assistive devices
  availability of, 58
  as factor in falls, 16, 19, 42
  intervention strategies, 88
  memory/cognitive impaired care recipients, 91
  Morse Fall Scale, 68, 69
  safety checklist, 89
  VA fall reduction programs, 139

B

Balancing measures, 118
Bar graphs, 121, 122
Bathroom intervention strategies, 39, 41, 88
Bed alarms
  as factor in falls, 32
  intervention strategies, 40, 41, 91
Bed rails
  alternative to, 46
  as factor in falls, 16, 45
  intervention strategies, 40, 41, 45, 87
  use of, 40
Beds
  intervention strategies, 40, 41, 44–45, 87, 91
  position of, 40, 55, 57
  safety checklist, 89
  VA fall reduction programs, 140
Behavioral health care organizations medication assessment and reassessment, 36–37
Benchmarking
  assessment tools for, 8
  availability of data, 8
  fall definition and, 14, 121–122
  fall rates, 121–22
Biotechnology managers, 53, 54
Blame and shame culture, 3

C

CAHPS (Consumer Assessment of Health Plans), 8
Care planning and provision
  individual-specific interventions, 44, 55, 57–58, 61
  intervention strategies, 33, 41–45
  risk factor knowledge and, 104
  as root cause of falls, 30, 32
  staff communication, 32, 64
  timely care, 29, 30, 45
Care recipients
  definition, 4
  individual-specific interventions, 99–100
    bed rails, 87
    care planning and provision, 44, 55, 57–58, 61
    environment of care, 58, 87–88, 89
    gait and mobility problems, 92–94
    high-risk care recipients, 91–94
    home care organizations, 58
    long term care organizations, 58
    memory/cognitive impaired care recipients, 91
  safety measures for, 83–84
  transfer protocols, 94–99, 100, 101
  trends by population, 58
Case studies
  acute care fall reduction program, 142
  Morton Plant Mease Health Care (MPMHC) medication review process, 43–44
  Northeast Health System fall reduction program, 112–14
  nursing home fall reduction program, 142
  residential care fall reduction program, 141
  subacute fall reduction program, 141
  Umeå University Hospital, Sweden, stroke patient fall prediction index, 70–78
  unit-specific fall reduction programs, 105–110
  VA fall reduction programs, 138–140, 143
  VA reduction of restraint use project, 46–49
Categories of falls
  data analysis, 121, 122
  intrinsic/extrinsic risk factors, 16
  Morse Fall Scale, 15–16, 67–69, 84, 86
Causes of falls. *See* Risk factors
CDC. *See* Centers for Disease Control and Prevention (CDC)
Centers for Disease Control and Prevention (CDC)
  common causes of falls, 19
  Falls in Nursing Homes Fact Sheet, 15
  fall statistics, 14–15, 20–22
Central nervous system disorders, 19
Changing Approach to Falls in the Elderly (Steinweg), 16–17
Checklists
  accident/incident investigation form, 111
  fall risks, 39, 40
  physical assessment after a fall, 55, 56
  postfall checklists, 55, 56, 57
Chronic care measures, 136–137
Clinical nurse specialist (CNS), 115
Clinical practice guidelines, 55, 83, 84
Cognitive/memory problem interventions, 44, 91
Communication issues
  in care planning and provision, 32, 64
  intervention strategies, 32–33
  as root cause of falls, 30, 31
  staffing levels, concerns about, 34–35

Comprehensive medical assessments, 65, 66
Consumer Assessment of Health Plans (CAHPS), 8
Cost of falls
 financial cost, 21–22
 physical cost, 21
Critical access hospitals
 assessment for medication-induced falls, 25
 fall risk reduction (National Patient Safety Goal 9), 2
 fall risk reduction program requirement, 25
Culture of safety. *See* safety culture

D

Data analysis
 bar graphs, 121, 122
 fall rate, 119, 120–22
 injury rate, 119
 to reduce falls, 124–26
 run charts, 120
 standards
  changes based on data analysis (PI.3.10), 23, 130
  data analysis (PI.2.10), 129
  pattern and trend analysis (PI.2.20), 23, 129
  staffing effectiveness (HR.1.30) standard, 131–32, 133–37
 trends in falls, 119–20, 122–23
Data collection
 on fall occurrences, 82–83
 for interventions development, 104–5
 to measure program success, 118–19
 minimum data set (MDS) requirements, 124
 procedures for, 10
 standards
  data collection standard (PI.1.10), 23, 127–28
  staffing effectiveness (HR.1.30) standard, 131–32, 133–37
 unit-specific data, 105
Dementia, 38
Documentation
 fall risk in medical records, 33, 84
 forms and policies for, 105, 110–12
Downtown Index, 70
Dynamic Gait Index, 66

E

Education. *See* patient and family education; staff education and training
"Enhancing the Safety of Hospitalization by Reducing Patient Falls" (Morse), 112
Environment of care
 checklists to identify fall risks, 39, 40
 as factor in falls, 16, 18, 19
 Goal 9, National Patient Safety Goals, 25
 individual-specific interventions, 58, 87–88, 89
 intervention strategies, 38–41
 medical equipment safety checklist, 88, 89
 as root cause of falls, 30, 32
Ergonomics process, 96–97, 99, 102–103
Evidence of Standards Compliance, 25
Extrinsic risk factors, 16, 18

F

Facility managers, 53, 54
Fall Assessment Questionnaire (FAQ), 70
Fall cause analysis tool, 58, 60
Fall evaluations, 61
Fall-focused pharmaceutical intervention program (FFPIP), 43–44
"Fall Prediction Index for Patients in Stroke Rehabilitation" (Nyberg and Gustafson), 70
Fall prediction index for stroke patients, 70–78
Fall rates, 119, 120–122, 123
Fall reduction committee, 58
Fall reduction programs
 assessment process, importance of, 51–52
 challenges of, 13
 effectiveness measurement, 117–120
 example of, 81–82
 forms and policies for, 105, 110–112
 Goal 9, National Patient Safety Goals, 25
 implementation of, 140
 institutional support for, 112, 115, 132, 140
 monitoring of, 84
 monitoring systems, 123
 Northeast Health System fall reduction program, 112–114
 principles of, 82–84
 process to reduce falls, 83
 staff education and training on, 84
 unit-specific fall reduction programs, 105–110
 VA fall reduction programs, 138–140, 143

Fall risk reduction
clinical practice guidelines, 55, 83, 84
National Patient Safety Goal 9
applicability of, 2
goals of, 2, 25
requirements for, 25
patient and family education on, 37, 64
Fall risk scores, 58, 59
Falls
definitions, 14
frequency of, 13, 14–15
impact of, 1
predictability of, 52
Falls and Fall Risk Clinical Practice Guidelines (AMDA), 55, 83, 84
Falls clinical nurse specialist, 53
Falls in Nursing Homes Fact Sheet (CDC), 15
Fear of falling, 63–64
FFPIP (fall-focused pharmaceutical intervention program), 43–44
Financial cost of falls, 21–22
FOCUS-PDCA process, 106
Footwear
as factor in falls, 16, 19
intervention strategies, 88
Forms and policies for intervention documentation, 105, 110–112
Frequency of falls, 13, 14–15
Functional assessments, 55, 65, 66

G

Gait and mobility problems
as factor in falls, 16, 17, 19
functional assessment for, 66
intervention strategies, 92–94
Morse Fall Scale, 68, 69
quality indicators, 92–93
Geriatric assessments, 65
Geriatricians, 65, 66
Get Up and Go Test, 61, 66
Grading criteria for intervention strategies, 103–104

H

Hallway intervention strategies, 40, 88
Handrail intervention strategies, 40, 41
Health Plan Employer Data and Information Set (HEDIS), 8
Hendrich Fall Risk Model, 66
High-risk care recipients
individual-specific interventions, 91–94
unit-specific fall reduction programs, 105–110
Hip fractures, 20, 22
Hip protectors, 91
Home care organizations
assessment for medication-induced falls, 25
extrinsic fall risk factors, 18
fall incident evaluations, 82–83
fall risk reduction (National Patient Safety Goal 9), 2, 25
functional assessments, 66
individual-specific interventions, 58
medication errors, 18
sentinel event, falls as, 15
Hospital Bed Safety Workgroup, 45
"Hospital Report 2002" (Ontario Hospital Association), 8
Hospitals
acute care fall reduction program, 142
assessment for medication-induced falls, 25
fall rates, 122
fall risk reduction (National Patient Safety Goal 9), 2, 25
nursing assessments, 65–66
screening indicators, 134–135
sentinel event, falls as, 15
subacute fall reduction program, 141

I

I Hate Falling (mnemonic), 20
Illnesses as fall factor, 16, 17–18, 19, 62
Improving Organization Performance (PI)
standards, 126–27
changes based on data analysis (PI.3.10), 23, 130
data analysis (PI.2.10), 129
data collection (PI.1.10), 23, 127–128
pattern and trend analysis (PI.2.20), 23, 129
proactive process for safety risks (PI.3.20), 130–131
sentinel events management process (PI.2.30), 23, 129–130
Incident/accident investigation form, 111
Individual-specific interventions, 99–100
bed rails, 87
care planning and provision, 44, 55, 57–58, 61

environment of care, 58, 87–88, 89
gait and mobility problems, 92–94
high-risk care recipients, 91–94
home care organizations, 58
long term care organizations, 58
memory/cognitive impaired care recipients, 91
Injurious falls, 21, 118
Injury rate, 119
Institute of Medicine, 3
Interdisciplinary fall team, 52–61
Intervention strategies. *See also* Individual-specific interventions
assessment and reassessment, 35–38
bathrooms, 39, 41
bed alarms, 40, 41
bed rails, 40, 45
beds, 40, 44–45
care planning, 33, 41–45
communication issues, 32–33
data collection for, 104–105
environment of care, 38–41
floor surfaces, 40
grading criteria, 103–104
hallways, 40
handrails, 40, 41
hip protectors, 91
institutional support for, 112, 115, 132, 140
lighting issues, 40
memory/cognitive problem interventions, 44, 91
principles of, 84–87
purpose of, 87
research-based decision-making and interventions, 100–101, 103–104
restraint use, 40, 45
result-oriented interventions, 85
staff education and training, 33–35
Intrinsic risk factors, 16–18

J

Joint Commission
safety culture assessments requirements, 1
sentinel event, falls as, 15, 22–23
Sentinel Event Advisory Group, 23–24
Sentinel Event Database, 23
Sentinel Event Policy, 23

L

Liability claims for falls, 22, 23
Licensed practical nurses (LPNs), 53, 54
Lifting patients. *See* Transfer protocols
Lighting issues
as factor in falls, 16, 18
intervention strategies, 40
Long term care organizations
assessment for medication-induced falls, 25
assessment to determine transfer method, 95
causes of falls in, 15, 52
comprehensive medical assessments, 65
data collection (PI.1.10), 23, 128
fall rates, 122
fall risk reduction (National Patient Safety Goal 9), 2, 25
fall statistics, 15
individual-specific interventions, 58
nursing assessments, 65–66
nursing home fall reduction program, 142
screening indicators, 136
sentinel event, falls as, 15
LPNs (licensed practical nurses), 53, 54

M

Malpractice claims for falls, 22, 23
Management of Human Resources staffing effectiveness (HR.1.30) standard, 131–132, 133–137
Management self-assessment tools, 5–6
Medical assessments, 65, 66
Medical equipment
for patient transfers and lifting, 95–96
preventive maintenance program, 39, 40
safety checklist, 88, 89
Medical patients, 58
Medical record documentation, 33, 84
Medication issues
assessment and reassessment, 25, 36–38, 41, 42, 64–65
errors in home care settings, 18
as factor in falls, 16, 18, 19, 24–25
medications that predispose falls, 21, 43
pharmacists' role in fall reduction, 42–44
VA fall reduction programs, 139
Medication reconciliation (National Patient Safety Goal 8)
compliance suggestions, 90

goals and requirements, 24–25
rehabilitation center medication review process, 43–44
Memory/cognitive problem interventions, 44, 91
Mental status
as factor in falls, 16, 19
Morse Fall Scale, 68, 69
Minimum data set (MDS) requirements, 124
Mnemonic for physical findings in elderly people, 19, 20
Mobility aids. *See* Assistive devices
Mobility problems. *See* Gait and mobility problems
Monitoring systems, 123
Morse Fall Scale, 15–16, 66, 67–69
Morse Risk Assessment Tool, 67–69
Morton Plant Mease Health Care (MPMHC), 43–44
Musculoskeletal disorder (MSD), 96

N

National Center for Patient Safety (NCPS) Falls Toolkit
care recipient assessment, 90–91
environment of care interventions, 87–88
gait and mobility problem interventions, 93–94
interdisciplinary fall team, 53
memory/cognitive problem interventions, 91
program effectiveness measurement, 117–120
National Committee for Quality Assurance, Quality Compass, 8
National Patient Safety Goals
applicability of, 24
basis for, 23
compliance evaluation, 23, 25
fall risk reduction (Goal 9)
applicability of, 2
goals of, 2, 25
requirements for, 25
medication reconciliation (Goal 8)
compliance suggestions, 90
goals and requirements, 24–25
rehabilitation center medication review process, 43–44
program-specific nature of, 24
NCPS. *See* National Center for Patient Safety (NCPS) Falls Toolkit
Nonpunitive culture promotion, 5–6
Northeast Health System fall reduction program, 112–114
Nurse managers, 53, 54
Nurse practitioners, 53, 54
Nursing assessments, 65–66
Nursing assistants, 53, 54
Nursing home fall reduction program, 142
Nursing home resident screening indicators, 137

O

Occupational Safety & Health Administration (OSHA)
ergonomics process, 97, 99, 102–103
staff safety in care recipient transfers, 94
transfer protocols, 96
applicability of methods, 95
lateral transfers, 98
repositioning in bed, 99
repositioning in chair, 100
seated positions, 97
up from floor, 101
Occupational therapists, 53, 54
Ontario Hospital Association, "Hospital Report 2002", 8
Organization cultures
assessment of, 3–4
intervention strategies support, 112, 115, 132, 140
nonpunitive culture promotion, 5–6
as root cause of falls, 30, 32
transformation to safer care, 3
OSHA. *See* Occupational Safety & Health Administration (OSHA)
Osteoporotic fractures, 22
Outcome measures, 118
Outpatient setting assessments, 65

P

Pathological culture, 3
Pathologic conditions contributing to falls, 17
Patient, 4. *See also* Care recipients
Patient and family education, 37, 64
Patient safety managers, 53, 54
Patient safety programs, 7–8
Pattern and trend analysis (PI.2.20), 23, 129
Performance improvement process, 126–127
Periodic Performance Review (PPR), 25
Pharmacists
as members of fall reduction team, 53, 54
role in fall reduction program, 42–44

Physical assessment after a fall, 55, 56
Physical cost of falls, 21
Physical environment. *See* environment of care
Physical therapists, 53, 54, 66
Physicians, 53, 54
Physiologic falls
  anticipated physiologic falls
    definition, 15, 67–68
    frequency of, 15
    intervention strategies, 86
    precautionary strategies, 86
  unanticipated physiologic falls
    definition, 15, 67
    frequency of, 15
    intervention strategies, 86
Physiology of falls, 34
Plan-Do-Study-Act (PDSA) process, 8
Polypharmacy, 25, 34
Post-acute care measures, 137
Postfall assessments, 65
Postfall checklists, 55, 56, 57
Precautionary strategies for anticipated falls, 86
Predictive scales for fall risks, 87
Previous falls, 16
Proactive process for safety risks (PI.3.20), 130–131
Process measures, 118
Protective strategies, 86–87
Psychiatric patients, 58

Q

Quality Compass (National Committee for Quality Assurance), 8
Quality improvement, risk analysis for, 82, 83
"Quality Indicators for the Management and Prevention of Falls and Mobility Problems in Vulnerable Elders" (Rubenstein), 92–93
Quality management coordinators, 53, 54

R

Reassessment. *See* assessment and reassessment
Rehabilitation centers
  fall rates, 122
  medication review process, 43–44
Reporting methods, 14
Repositioning patients. *See* Transfer protocols
Research-based decision-making and interventions, 100–101, 103–104
Resident, 4. *See also* Care recipients
Residential care fall reduction program, 141
Restraint use
  as factor in falls, 16, 19
  intervention strategies, 40, 45
  reduction of use and alternatives to, 46–49
  VA reduction of restraint use project, 46–49
Result-oriented interventions, 85
Risk analysis of falls, 82, 83
Risk assessment. *See* Assessment and reassessment
Risk factors, 16, 52
  assistive devices, 16, 19
  central nervous system disorders, 19
  common causes, 18–19
  data analysis, 121, 122
  environment of care, 16, 18, 19
  extrinsic, 16, 18
  fear of falling, 63–64
  footwear, 16, 19
  gait issues, 16, 17, 19
  illnesses, 16, 17–18, 19, 62
  injurious falls, 21
  intrinsic, 16–18
  lighting issues, 16, 18
  medication issues, 16, 18, 19, 21, 24–25
  mental status, 16, 19
  mnemonic for physical findings, 19, 20
  multiple, 62–64
  pathologic conditions, 17
  predictive scales for, 87
  restraint use, 16, 19
  strokes, 62
  vision and visual abilities, 16, 17, 19
"Risk Factors for Falls of Hospitalized Stroke Patients" (Tutuarimia, van Straten, and Limburg), 62
Root causes analysis, 58, 60
Root causes of falls, 30–32
Run charts, 120

S

Safe Medication Use Expert Committee (U.S. Pharmacopeia), 18
Safety culture
  benefits of, 1
  challenges to, 3
  characteristics of, 3
  definition, 5

identification of problems in, 7
improvement of, 11-12
interest in, 1-2
nonpunitive culture promotion, 5-6
proactive process for safety risks (PI.3.20), 130-131
"Safety Culture Assessment" (Nieva and Sorra), 3, 5-12
Safety culture assessments
implementation of, 7
Joint Commission requirements for, 1
purpose of, 1-2
reasons to conduct, 7-8
Safety culture assessment tools
availability of, 9
changes based on, 11-12
characteristics of, 5-6
development of, 6, 12
procedures for use, 10
quality of, 9
reviews of, 10
selection of, 8-10
Safety measures for care recipients, 83-84
Screening indicators, 132, 134-137
Sentinel Event Advisory Group (Joint Commission), 23-24
Sentinel Event Database (Joint Commission), 23
Sentinel Event Policy (Joint Commission), 23
Sentinel events
definition, 23
falls as, 15, 22-23
Joint Commission standards for, 23, 129-130
organization-specific definition of, 23
response to, 23
sentinel events management process (PI.2.30), 23, 129-130
Stability, age-related factors, 17
Staff-based assessment tools, 6
Staff education and training
assessment and reassessment, 61
fall reduction programs, 34, 84, 140
fall risk factors, 34
Goal 9, National Patient Safety Goals, 25
intervention strategies, 33-35
physiology of falls, 34
as root cause of falls, 30, 31
unsafe conditions, 32
Staffing effectiveness (HR.1.30) standard, 131-132, 133-137
Staffing levels
communication of concerns about, 34-35
importance of, 32
as root cause of falls, 30, 31
Staff issues
communication issues, 30, 31, 64
ergonomics process, 96-97, 99, 102-103
as members of fall reduction team, 53-54
transfer protocol safety, 94
work-related injuries, 94, 96-97, 99, 102-103
Statistics on falls, 13, 14-15
financial cost of falls, 21-22
physical cost of falls, 21
strokes as risk factor, 62
Strategies for Leadership (VHA and AHA), 5
STRATIFY model, 66
Stroke patients
assessment tools, 70
fall prediction index, 70-78
risk factors for, 62
Subacute fall reduction program, 141
Success of fall reduction programs, 117-120
Sundowning, 38
Supply procurement and distribution managers, 53, 54
Surgical patients, 58

T

TCU (transitional care unit) fall reduction programs, 105-110
Team approach to assessment, 36, 51, 52-54
Timed Get Up and Go Test, 66
Tinetti Performance Oriented Mobility Assessment, 66
Toileting schedules, 44, 45, 86, 91, 121
VA fall reduction programs, 139
Transfer protocols
applicability of methods, 95
assessment to determine transfer method, 94-95
care recipient safety, 94
equipment selection, 95-96
Goal 9, National Patient Safety Goals, 25
Occupational Safety & Health Administration (OSHA), 96
lateral transfers, 98
repositioning in bed, 99
repositioning in chair, 100
seated positions, 97
up from floor, 101

staff safety, 94
Transitional care unit (TCU) fall reduction programs, 105–10
Transportation managers, 53, 54
Traumatic brain injuries (TBI), 20–21
Trends in falls
care recipients, 58
data analysis, 119–120, 122–123
pattern and trend analysis (PI.2.20), 23, 129
unit-specific fall trends, 122–123

U

Umeå University Hospital, Sweden, stroke patient fall prediction index, 70–78
Unanticipated physiologic falls
definition, 15, 67
frequency of, 15
intervention strategies, 86
Unit-specific data, 105
Unit-specific fall reduction programs, 105–110
Unit-specific fall trends, 122–123
University of Texas safety culture assessment, 6
Unwitnessed falls, 118
U.S. Department of Labor, Occupational Safety & Health Administration (OSHA). *See* Occupational Safety & Health Administration (OSHA)
U.S. Department of Veterans Affairs (VA). *See also* U.S. Veterans Health Administration (VHA)
fall reduction programs, 138–140, 143
restraint use reduction and alternatives, 46–49
U.S. Pharmacopeia Safe Medication Use Expert Committee, 18
U.S. Veterans Health Administration (VHA)
National Center for Patient Safety (NCPS)
Falls Toolkit
care recipient assessment, 90–91
environment of care interventions, 87–88
gait and mobility problem interventions, 93–94
interdisciplinary fall team, 53
memory/cognitive problem interventions, 91
program effectiveness measurement, 117–120
safety culture assessment, 6

V

VA. *See* U.S. Department of Veterans Affairs (VA)
VHA (Voluntary Hospitals of America), *Strategies for Leadership*, 5
Vision and visual abilities as factor in falls, 16, 17, 19

W

Work-related injuries, 94, 96–97, 99, 102–103

Other Joint Commission Resources Titles of Interest

Title	Order Code and ISBN	Price
Patient Safety Essentials for Health Care: Third Edition This book includes all Joint Commission standards, rationales, elements of performance, and scoring information that relate to patient safety. Commonalities among the standards are addressed so that readers understand which standards apply to which settings.	**PSE-03** (ISBN: 0-86688-901-9)	$75.00
The Joint Commission Guide to Priority Focus Areas This handy book is an all-in-one source on the Priority Focus Areas (PFAs), a part of the Joint Commission's new accreditation process.	**PFA-04** (ISBN: 0-86688-841-1)	$70.00
The Physician's Promise: Protecting Patients from Harm This exception book approaches the patient safety initiative from the perspective of physicians, and addresses workload, time constraints, and communication issues.	**PPPH-02** (ISBN: 0-86688-798-9)	$55.00
What Every Health Care Organization Should Know About Sentinel Events The most prevalent sentinel events and where they occur are discussed in this book, with explanations on the need for adverse event reporting and pinpointing causes, so that high risk activities and populations can be identified before a sentinel event occurs.	**HSE-200** (ISBN: 0-86688-911-6)	$75.00

Joint Commission Newsletters	Online Only	Online and Print
Joint Commission Perspectives on Patient Safety™		
U.S.	$249	$299
Canada or Mexico	$249	$350
International	$249	$389
Environment of Care® News		
U.S.	$249	$299
Canada or Mexico	$249	$344
International	$249	$389
Joint Commission Benchmark®		
U.S.	$145	$180
Canada or Mexico	$145	$220
International	$145	$234

Ways to Order

1. ONLINE: http://www.jcrinc.com.
2. PHONE: To place your credit card order by phone, call our Customer Service Center toll free at 877/223-6866 (8 A.M.-8 P.M. central standard time).
3. NEWSLETTERS: Call our Customer Service Center toll free at 800/346-0085 ext. 9558.

Phone or online orders may be paid with a Visa, MasterCard, or American Express Card.